That One Shower

"I cautiously raised my hands to my head, antici-pating what exactly would happen when I massaged the conditioner through my hair. In a matter of seconds, as I glimpsed down at my trembling hands, I noticed two handfuls of hair that had completely fallen out. I collapsed onto the frigid bathtub surface, hysterically crying in dismay. Everything merged into a colossal blur. The water from the showerhead above me, and my tears mingled together, making it impossible to see, and impossible for me to wrap my head around the fact that I was losing my hair…all of it."

FALLING OUT

Losing Hair, Gaining Confidence

By Lesley Minervini

Library of Congress Cataloging-in-Publication Data

Minervini, Lesley
    Falling Out/Lesley Minervini
      p. cm.
    ISBN 978-0-9829676-5-2
    1. Health, Mind & Body - Disorders
    2. Teens - Health, Mind & Body
    3. Health, Mind & Body - Beauty & Fashion

This publication is designed to provide accurate and authoritative information in regard to the subject matter covered. It is sold with the understanding that neither the author nor the publisher is registered experts in the subject matter discussed. If legal advice or other expert assistance is required, the services of a competent professional person should be sought.

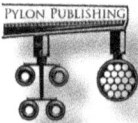

Attention: Hospitals, Schools, and Businesses

www.pylonpublishing.com

Pylon Publishing books are available at quantity discounts with bulk purchase for educational, business, or sales promotional use. For information go to www.pylonpublishing.com

Contents

Dedication... 7

Special Thanks.. 9

Poem- Sorry I'm Not…... 11

Chapter One- Like Mother, Like Daughter............. 13

Chapter Two- The Bald and the Beautiful............... 21

Chapter Three- Alo…Ar…WHAT?!......................... 29

Chapter Four- Army Attack at Lunch...................... 39

Chapter Five- Never Trust a Hat.............................. 49

Chapter Six- I Finally Have Barbie™ Hair................. 59

Chapter Seven- Can You Hold This Please?............ 71

Chapter Eight- For You, Lord.................................. 83

Chapter Nine- The Real Deal................................... 93

Chapter Ten- It's Okay, Everything's Okay............... 103

Contact Information.. 113

Dedication

Dominic Drumright and Luke Drumright,

You two boys deserve this book and the lessons included in it. I only hope I inspired you both to live your lives to the fullest, and to rock on with or without hair. Because you guys have definitely inspired me. I love you both so much!

Special Thanks

Sara Davenport—I can't even begin to thank you for all of this. Without you, my experiences would not have developed into an actual book, a real story. You are way more than a co-author to me; you have become an everlasting friend and I could not ask for more than that.

Dawn Young—The one who started it all! You told me that I have this disease for a reason, and God was telling me something needed to be done…a book perhaps? I love you and thank you for pushing me into writing this.

My family—My true backbone. I would not be where I am today without any of you. Your unconditional love and support gives me the opportunity to stay positive and determined through every obstacle. I love each and every one of you.

Catherine Arend—You have been by my side, through thick and thin, ever since we met. You never give up on me, and you always steer me towards the right path. You are my miracle, Miss C. I love you with all my heart.

_____, You definitely know who you
_{Friends, insert your name here}
are! I cannot thank you enough for everything you've done for me. Your constant support and encouraging words keep me strong and optimistic. Thanks so much for the laughter, the hugs, the tears, and the love.

Xoxo,
Lesley

Sorry I'm Not...

Sorry I'm not skinny; I'm proud of my curves.
Sorry my hair isn't gorgeous; I'm proud to wear a wig.
Sorry if I'm too upfront; I'm proud to speak my mind.
Sorry I don't lie to make it hurt less; I'm proud to be honest.
Sorry I'm not easy; I'm proud of my morals.
Sorry that I'm jealous; I'm proud to be protective.
Sorry I'm not perfect; I'm proud of my flaws.
Sorry I'm not who you want me to be; I'm proud to be myself.

Like Mother, Like Daughter

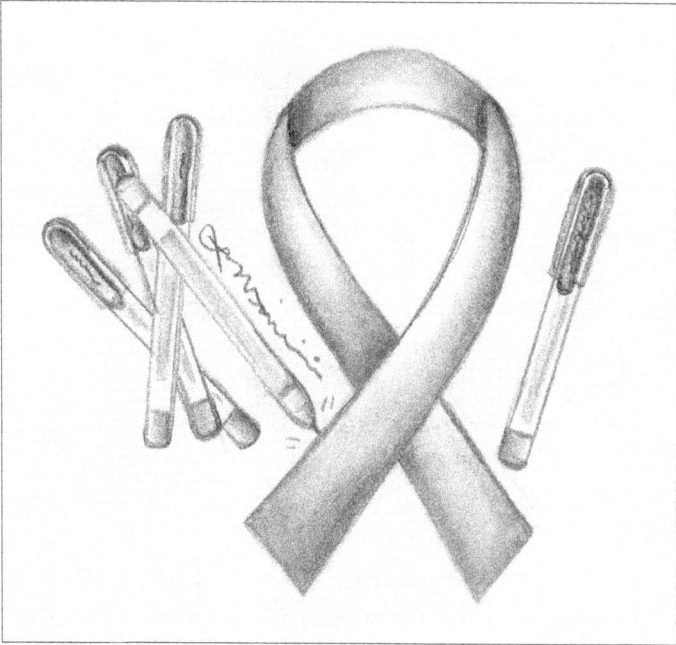

"Lesley, you my dear, are just like your mommy...a saint."

~Courtney J.

I quickly opened my eyes, staring at the white, blank ceiling above me that eventually brought me back to reality from my fairytale dreams as a seven-year-old. I lay there motionless, remembering that my birthday was getting close. Soon after, I smiled to myself, realizing close meant that it was in less than a month. I flew out of bed and ran down the short hallway to my staircase. I clutched the knob of the banister pole and positioned myself to swing frantically around it like I always did. But something stopped me that morning...

My parent's bedroom is directly across from the stairs, so it's a clear view in from where I was standing. Both of them were sitting on the edge of the bed; my mom had her left arm up awkwardly above her head, and my dad seemed to be examining something under it. They were conversing quietly to one another which just sounded like mumbling to me.

"Dad?" I interrupted.

"Hi, Les." He said without turning his head from my mother.

"What are you doing?" I asked, playing the predictable role of the obnoxious child constantly asking questions.

My mom finally looked over at me. I had always thought she was beautiful. She has mid-length, thin brown hair that she spends what seems to be hours on, in order to create "some volume." Her gentle, hazel eyes, her pale skin, and her warm smile cause anyone she approaches to feel 100 percent comfortable in her presence. You need to understand just how important my mom really is in my life. My brother Michael and I come first, for both my parents actually. Even though we are complete opposites of each other, my brother and I are still their babies, their angels.

Her main focus is to help others. Let me give you an example. One day my mom had picked me up from Bradford Primary School, and as we drove through the famous four-way-stop of Valley Parkway and Club Drive, she saw a kid get hit by a bus directly behind us. In a matter of seconds she had pulled over, put the car in park, and darted out of the vehicle towards the intersection. She had ordered me to stay right there in the car. My neighborhood friend Christina Munson was with me, so we glimpsed at each other, unbuckled our seatbelts, and turned around swiftly to observe the chaotic situation occurring behind us.

My mom sprinted towards the scene of the stopped big yellow bus and the small boy below it. He had started to cross the street when the bus, not noticing him, continued to make its right turn. The boy fell into the wheel but fortunately was knocked backwards. Miraculously, the boy walked away with only a cut up elbow. A few other cars had stopped along the roads, and people started to cluster together so they could share perspectives about the accident. My mom was still over at the corner where it happened, now with both Principals from Bradford Primary and Intermediate. They had been called immediately and came down to investigate and help out.

Suddenly a car abruptly parked, practically in the middle of the intersection, and a woman flew out of the driver's side, imitating almost the exact actions of my mom. Her face was clouded with concern, extremely pale with tears streaming down her face. She bolted across to the corner where the boy was and literally threw herself upon him, picking him up, and holding him so tightly I thought she might break him in half. She rocked him in her arms back and forth as she sat on the edge of the sidewalk curb; it was his mom.

Finally, my mom started back to the car, in a much calmer fashion. Christina and I sat speechless. We didn't really have to ask what happened, but I could sense her frustration with all of it. She said she had spoken to the Principals, explaining how dangerous the four-way-stop was when kids tried to walk home from school. The principals simply stated they couldn't really do anything about it. Instead, my mom said she would.

Shortly after, my mom and her good friend, Michelle Arend, brought together a handful of moms that lived back in Ken Caryl Valley, where we lived, to be included in a system called "The Crossing Guard". My friends and I knew them as the "crossing guard ladies," and they'd be at the four-way stop after school, wearing bright orange vests and holding bold red stop signs. They'd walk out in the middle of the intersection, make the cars stop, and tell the kids when to cross. Honestly, we all thought they were magic or something. There was no doubt in my heart of her devotion to this issue and the determination she possessed to fix it. That's my mom!

As she looked over at me from her bedroom that morning, her eyes were wide and her mouth was partially open as she searched for the words to use.

"Well sweetie, it looks like we found some sort of a lump right here that the doctor may have to check out." She pointed somewhat to her left armpit.

"Oh. Well okay." I turned and dashed down the stairs, anticipating some delicious breakfast in the kitchen which seemed much more appealing to me than a lump on an armpit. Both my parents had acted so calm upstairs that I didn't worry about it. The concern of her going to the doctors began fading from my thoughts until October 7, 1999, when my mom, Jody Minervini, was diagnosed with breast cancer.

* * *

"Chemo what?"

"Chemotherapy Lesley," my dad said. "That's what's going to help mom get better. But this is going to make her lose all of her hair…that's what the medicine does. But she'll be okay honey, I promise."

As a first grader, I didn't understand any of this whatsoever. I knew that cancer was a "bad thing," but breast cancer? Was that really scary or something? My parents seemed so undisturbed about the whole situation that it allowed me not to worry, not to get caught up in all of it. I guess I knew she was sick. However, I didn't comprehend the chance of her dying. I didn't understand the whole life and death situation. She was too strong in my little perfect world for something like that to happen; she was invincible in my eyes. I noticed adults like my teachers, my friends' parents, and my relatives growing more and more concerned; they seemed so serious about it all. But she still seemed fine to me, so I was okay.

The night Mom got home from her first treatment of chemotherapy, she brought me upstairs to her bathroom. I absolutely loved that room; it was so spacious yet isolated from the rest of the house. It had gigantic mirrors all around, so I easily amused myself. She grabbed some small scissors out of her drawer. They were the ones she'd use to cut me or Michael's hair when it seemed necessary. They were tiny, but keen-edged, and had white rubber grips around the finger holes.

"So because mommy's going to lose her hair soon, I think we should cut it really short…so it's easier when it starts falling out. You want to?!" She gazed at me, almost excited to ask me this. She was smiling, of course, and made me feel comfortable.

"Sure!" I replied.

She handed the scissors over to me carefully, and told me to go for it. She was sitting with her legs crossed on the edge of the bathtub, and I was balancing above her on the platform behind it. An elementary age girl, cutting off all of her mother's hair in front of the mirror: you don't see that every day. She had put all trust in me, all control. And I accepted it. I took a deep breath, gently grabbed a piece of her brown thin hair, raised the scissors to it, and cut about seven to ten inches off. I held it in my hand for a minute and just thought about how different her hair was from mine.

I was suddenly aware of my own hair. Up until then, it was just a hassle to untangle every morning. Now I took notice of how thick mine was compared to her fine hair. And it was so jet black next to her soft brown shade. I hadn't really ever cared for it before, but I was suddenly grateful for every strand on my head. I let go of the piece of her hair and grabbed another patch, cutting off the same amount. I'd glance up at the mirror every once in a while to see her reaction. She was still smiling, much less now, but a vague grin rested on her face. I continued, feeling more and more confident in myself.

"Good job sweetie."

*   *   *

Later in the process of chemo, my family and I were sitting at the table eating dinner. When my mom started her chemo, we began to receive complete meals from close family friends, neighborhood folks, and relatives. Michael and I kind of enjoyed it; dinner was already prepared and usually tasty every night.

We all finished our meal, and I began drawing pictures at the kitchen table with my famous gel pens. I called them milky pens, and I probably had every single color possible. It got to a point where getting a single new milky pen was like getting a brand new puppy. My dad obviously recognized my obsession, and found it humorous to blurt out, "milky pens!!!!" whenever he discovered them. I remember slyly bringing them to the table, hoping he wouldn't notice. But before I could even set them down, he spotted them. I held my breath and just anxiously waited. He took a deep breath in, held it for a moment, and stared back at me, then shouted, "Milky pens!!!!" I fell into unstoppable laughter, and we all did the same. In spite of everything Mom was going through, my parents worked extremely hard to keep the family time as normal as they could.

My mom was completely bald by this point, which was the only give away to the struggle she was facing. To deal with it, she purchased a wig, but back then wigs were poorly made and fake looking, so she favored hats. She had taken her hat off at dinner that night. My brother and I were still a bit shocked by the pale, one colored scalp, but it didn't stop us from stuffing our faces.

Suddenly, my mom said that she wanted Michael and me to draw on her head with my milky pens. "What?!" I thought to myself. We hesitated, but once again, she had that excitement in her voice, so we took her up on the offer. I gave Michael a few gel pens (the ones I wasn't too fond of) and he walked to one side while I took the other. I remember her head being so smooth, so shiny, no hair there whatsoever. It seemed so vulnerable and fragile, I was almost scared to touch it let alone draw on it. But sure enough, we did. And the whole time all of us were giggling and smiling. My dad snapped pictures right and left, after every drawing had been finished. By the end of it, my mom's head looked like a collage of various kid masterpieces. She didn't need hair, she had gel pens, and she had us. I slowly stepped back to admire our artwork; it was amazing. As I stared, beaming, I had no idea I'd be in such a similar position. No one told me I'd be there in five years.

The Bald and the Beautiful

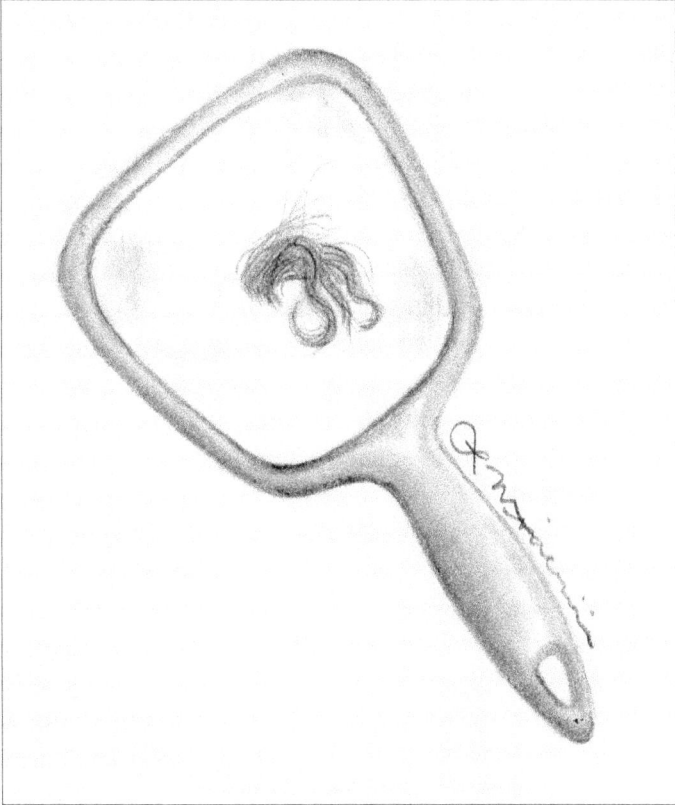

"You have an incredible and immeasurable amount
of strength and you are a fantastic writer. I know how
powerful a person you are… in all the low spots darlin',
I know you can pull yourself out."

~Dylan S.

I never thought I'd be much of a soap opera fan; during those mornings of groggy T.V. watching, occasionally, the channel would be playing a random soap opera. I never understood them completely. I mean, to me, it seemed like a bunch of pretty, yet depressed, actors who had the amazing talent of crying on demand. However, Michelle Arend (my mom's best friend), would drastically change my mind one summer. Michelle was basically my second mom and had been friends with my mom since I was a baby. It must be a generational thing because Catherine Arend, her daughter, was my best friend ever since we started creating our first words. They live one block away, so that always makes it easy to see each other and hang out whenever we feel it is necessary…And that seems to be every single day in the summertime.

The summer of 2005, though, was when Michelle had her real opportunity to convince Catherine and me, now official teenagers at thirteen, of the "true meaning" behind soap operas. It took her the entire morning to explain the whole drama and background of "The Bold and the Beautiful," but she accomplished the task, and Catherine and I were suddenly interested. We began watching the next episode that was on at noon, and both got comfortable on her parents' bed. Once I was settled, I ran my fingers through my hair as I relaxed, but instead I grew uneasy about something. I noticed a small, smooth, circular spot on the back of my head where there was absolutely no hair. I wasn't going to assume anything right away, but during a commercial I decided to ask Catherine about it.

"Hey Catherine, come look at this. I just felt it now." I slowly bent my head down and flipped over all of my hair to make the spot visible to her. I felt her kind of fingering through my hair and then gently touch the bald spot like she was somewhat startled by it.

Finally, after a while of investigating my scalp, Catherine said, "Umm, I'm not sure Les, I think you just have a weird hairline." I appreciated my best friend always trying to reassure me when the worst was about to happen, but I'm sure that both of us knew what was really happening, we were just too afraid to admit it. All of a sudden, we didn't need some silly soap opera for drama.

After being at her house the night before, Catherine slept over at my house after our discovery because we didn't want to be separated. Catherine knew I needed her for whatever this small bald spot may play out to be. The two of us did our best to focus on, and discuss, other things, but we were still both contemplating how this hair situation would affect me, and what it was in general.

The next morning, I knew I had to shower quickly because my family was supposed to go to church. Both of my parents, my mom especially, came from a Catholic background. My family is a mixture of Italian and Irish, so being baptized as a Catholic was definitely a necessity. I've been going to church for as long as I can remember. When my parents moved to Ken Caryl, they searched for a suitable Catholic church in the area, and finally found Saint Francis Cabrini. The church was only about 15 minutes away, which made it convenient to go every Sunday. I never dreaded church like a majority of little kids, but I didn't exactly understand the details and meaning of Mass yet. However, I did understand the peaceful, welcoming atmosphere, and I always felt pure joy being there.

*   *   *

I stepped in the shower, rinsed off my hair, and struggled to get the last bit of shampoo out of the bottle. As I scrubbed the bubbly substance all over my scalp, I felt a few strands of hair tangled around my fingers. "No big deal," I thought, "it's just a few hairs." Then, I actually looked at my hand; it was covered in a wad of my hair. I freaked myself out and quickly washed away the excess from my hand to feel like it never happened. I attempted to stay calm, at least to get through the rest of my shower and throw on a robe.

"Catherine?!" I yelled in a concerned tone towards the direction of my bedroom, where she was waiting for me to finish up.

"Catherine, come here. I think I lost even more hair in the shower…can you please come and check out that spot?" As I gazed in the large body mirror on my mom's closet door, out of the corner of my eye I saw Catherine rushing to where I stood frozen in front of the mirror. I began trying to somehow see the back of my head by turning and twisting into various directions, but I couldn't get a decent sight. I remembered that my dad's closet was directly across from it where another identical mirror was positioned; if I angled one of the mirror's in just the right spot, I could see the whole back of myself.

Catherine still stood next to me, looking in the mirror to try and see what I was seeing. I glanced over at her, her face tense and her eyes worried. I eventually moved the mirror to the exact angle, and lifted up my wet hair. It seemed to be heavier than anything at this point. Right along my bottom hairline, there was the bald spot. It almost glowed in the mirror the way it appeared to be so white in contrast with my black hair surrounding it. It was about the size of a golf ball, and extremely visible. Neither Catherine nor I spoke a word. After observing the spot in dismay, I finally reached up with my other hand and touched it: cold, smooth, and shiny. It reminded me of how my mother's head felt the night we drew on it with gel pens. Even though that had been five years ago, the memory suddenly flooded back to me.

"Les, I think you should tell your mom. After all, she is a nurse." Her words snapped me back into reality, and I took her simple advice. My mom was scurrying around the house, but I called for her to come upstairs. Already in the "running-around-zone," my mom swiftly ran up the stairs to her room where both Catherine I were still standing in front of the same mirror.

"Mom, look…I have like a bald spot back here." I turned my head to allow her to see it well. She gently ran her hand over it, noticing how smooth it was just like I had.

"When did you notice it, Lesley?" She asked.

"Well, yesterday Catherine and I found it, but then this morning in the shower, I think I lost more hair, so we looked at it again. I don't know what it is mom!" I began choking up on my last words, and tears flooded my eyes. I tried to keep them in by not blinking, but I couldn't help myself; I felt so scared and confused. Was I seriously losing some of my hair, for no reason whatso-ever? I didn't get it. As I broke down, my mom quickly grabbed me and brought me in close to her.

"Lesley, stop, it's going to be okay. I bet it's nothing

to get worked up about. We can go to the doctors, or we can ask Dawn about it. I promise it'll be okay." Dawn is our family hair stylist, but she is way more than that to us. She had been good friends and gone to school with my mom's sister Leslie (my name sake…Get it? Leslie? Lesley?).

I absolutely loved going to see Dawn; it was like a treat for me every time. She was always asking me about my friends and boys and whoever my new crush was at the time. And I loved sharing everything with her. I trusted Dawn from the very first appointment: not only with my hair, but also with my little secrets. She was loud and outgoing; there was never one awkward silence during the entire visit with her. Our conversations dominated all of the others in the salon as customers surrounding us would either join in or simply just listen to us. Dawn is gorgeous; she has the prettiest face with fun make-up, an edgy style, and her hair seems to be different somehow every time I see her. But I promise it always looks amazing on her. Dawn has four kids: two girls and two boys. She always has updated pictures of them for my mom and me to see. We enjoy observing how the four of them get older and continue to grow up.

One thing I admired most about Dawn was how optimistic she was no matter what the situation. She constantly made me laugh and smile, and not to mention, had the great talent of making my hair look fresh and beautiful. I looked up to her in a special kind of way, physically and mentally. I valued her fun, flirty style, but most importantly, her amount of positivity and love. The best part was that Dawn didn't even feel like an adult to me. Instead, she felt like one of my best friends or the older sister I never had. I definitely wanted to see her first about the hair crisis because I felt the most comfortable with her, and I bet she would figure it out. Through all of my experiences with Dawn, she made things better, and I only hoped that she would do the same with my hair issue.

"Hello beautiful!" Dawn shouted just as she finished with her previous client and ran over to me in the waiting room. I was so excited to see her and I jumped up and bolted across the waiting room obstacles to get to her. She sat me down at her station and right away began asking the ritual questions and updating me on the "411." I was so caught up in our conversations that I had completely forgotten about the bald spot.

Dawn had washed and rinsed my hair, and then began to comb through it. My hair had always been jet black, mostly straight with some wave, and very soft. As she brushed the back of my head, I saw her abruptly pause what she was doing. Finally she said,

"Lesley...did you know there was a bald spot back here?"

"Oh yeah, I totally forgot to tell you. It was one of the big questions we had for you this visit. My friend Catherine and I found it a couple days ago. Do you know what it is?" I watched Dawn as she closely examined the area.

"You know I hate to say this, but I think it might be a hair loss disease called Alopecia Areata (Al-o-pee-sha Air-ee-ah-ta)." The words sounded ridiculous to me, almost like a name made up or something. My mom joined in on the conversation and told her side of the story. Dawn explained a little bit more about the disease and she recommended that I see a dermatologist to confirm it, but I decided to tune out. All of that worry came rushing back into my mind, and I wasn't exactly sure how to process what they were saying. I just stared into the mirror, directly at myself, trying to imagine a Lesley with less hair. "Alopecia Areata," I thought to myself, "why'd you pick me?"

Alo...Ar...WHAT?!

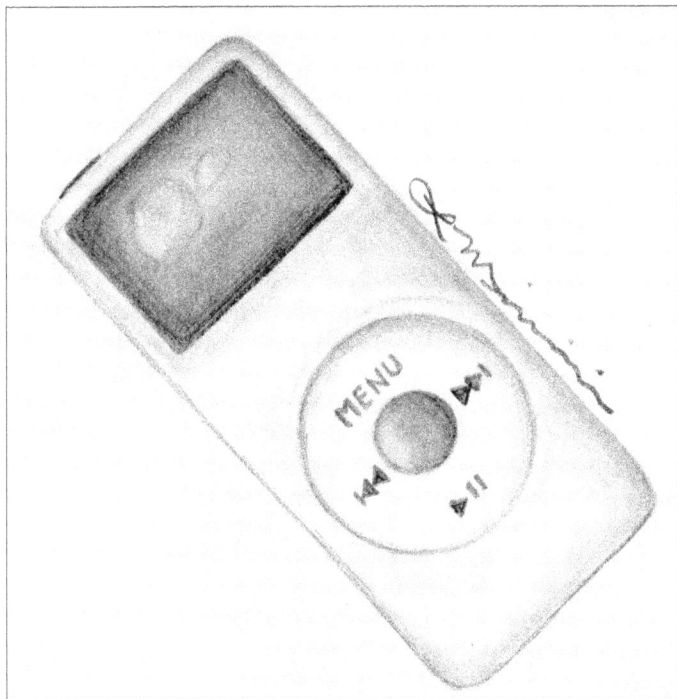

"Keep your head up, Gorgeous! You're still the prettiest
girl inside and out I've known since 4th grade!"
~Michaela S.

I had never been to a dermatologist before. Honestly, as a thirteen year old, I could barely pronounce the word. All I knew about it was that it focused on skin diseases, and all of my friends would go there for acne appointments and what not. But apparently, Alopecia was considered to be under a dermatologist's concerns. I wouldn't say I was actually afraid to go, I was definitely more curious. I had been so taken back by the first little bald spot on the back of my head that fear wasn't even able to conquer me yet. Instead, I kind of skipped that emotion for the time being, and moved on to looking for the real answers, and getting to the bottom of this.

My mom is the oldest of eight children, and comes from a big Catholic family: six girls and two boys. The sixth one born was my aunt, Leslie. Ironically, as her namesake, I resembled her more than any of my other aunts. I even took after some of her traits, like always creating a schedule and keeping things simple and organized. I loved her for that, and I was proud to follow in her footsteps.

Once my mom heard from Dawn that what I had could be a type of Alopecia, she automatically thought of Aunt Leslie. A couple years before, Aunt Leslie had noticed a small bald spot on the back of her head, just like I had. She eventually found Dr. S as her dermatologist who diagnosed her with Alopecia Areata. Dr. S's advice was to try Cortisone injections in the bald area. Aunt Leslie received the shots, saw hair re-growth within a month or so, and went on with her life like it had never happened. She had about three cycles with it, where she'd lose a small portion of hair in that same area, but once she went in for injections, her hair would slowly grow back with no problem.

After being told of Aunt Leslie's experience, I felt somewhat reassured and a bit more confident in seeing the dermatologist. My parents and I felt it would be best if I started out seeing the same doctor as Aunt Leslie because we already trusted her, and it seemed that almost everything that happened to Aunt Leslie would eventually happen to me; or at least that's how I liked to look at it.

It had been a couple of weeks since Catherine and I discovered my first spot, and unfortunately, I had lost just a little more hair. I now had two distinct bald spots, still located within the bottom layer of my hair, so they were easily out of sight to any surrounding people. Even though I made sure every morning both spots were completely covered up, I had this gut-wrenching feeling that they were somehow visible, or they were accidentally showing; I became paranoid. In school, I regularly began to sit in the back row of desks in each classroom, because I felt so self-conscious about a random person sitting behind me and observing the back of my head. And if I didn't get a back row desk in time, I remember having to sit in front of someone, and then spending the whole class thinking to myself that this stranger was full on staring at my head, burning a hole through it with his/her laser eyes. I couldn't stand it for much longer.

Basically, my mom's whole side of the family lived in and around Arvada. I loved having them all so close, it just made it that much easier to see and communicate with each other. Dr. S was located in Arvada also, so the drive was only about 20 to 30 minutes away from my house. As we drove there, I listened to various songs on my new "hot pink" iPod. That kept my mind off of everything for a bit longer, until we entered a series of dark brown, brick buildings. They didn't exactly look welcoming to me, and of course, the dermatologist's office was in one of them. I quickly shut off my iPod, rolled the earphones around it, and stuck it in my back pocket. My mom did her best to stay positive, like she always did, and she guided me into the building, through some hallways and directly to "Dermatology." She held the door open for me, watched me take a deep breath, and we walked in.

We waited in line and eventually reached the counter where we confirmed our appointment. I let my mom do the talking, because I still didn't understand fully all of the doctor appointments and paperwork and blah blah blah. I went and sat down and looked around the waiting room instead, where all sorts of people sat: some old, some young, some smiling, some frowning, some with company, and some alone. I had no idea a dermatologist's office could be this busy. I remember one old, fragile man, all by himself, with a large white bandage over one side of his forehead. I didn't want to stare (I had been taught that staring was rude), so I rapidly looked away and down at my hands. But I didn't focus on them, instead I thought of what was under that bandage. And not literally, but figuratively, like what experience was hiding itself under there? What pain, what sorrow, what suffering?

"Lesley?" the nurse's voice interrupted my thoughts. Both my mom and I hastily got up, smiled at the nurse so she knew it was us, and followed her through a long, narrow hallway to a room on the right side. Once all three of us were in the room, the nurse turned again and looked at my mom, then me, and said, "You're Miss Lesley, right?"

"Yeah," I nodded. She instructed me to sit down on

the "examination bed." I despised those things; they were the ones that had the thin, white paper along the top of them that would crinkle with every single move you made, even just breathing. I did my best to get situated up on it, and then stay frozen so I didn't have to hear the ridiculous crinkle of the tissue paper. My mom sat in a chair across from me, and then the nurse sat in another one at a desk with a computer. She swiveled towards me a little, with a booklet and pen in her hands, and began asking me some basic questions. They were nothing I hadn't heard before because they appeared to be regular physical check-up questions. It felt like we covered everything: my height, weight, allergies, asthma, eczema, pain, past medications, etc... Finally, she began asking more detailed questions relating to my hair loss. She asked to see the couple spots I had, so I flipped my hair over to show her. The nurse gently touched and rubbed both spots, just like Catherine and my mom had done. She stood silent for a while, but I sensed her observing each spot carefully.

"You can put your head back up now," the nurse said. She continued with her questions, "Now Lesley, do you get stressed very easily?"

I had no idea how that related to really anything, but I answered, "Well, kind of." Seventh grade was truly when I began pushing myself in school, and even other activities. I had always set high standards for myself, but they grew higher and higher as I entered each grade, getting closer to high school. I had gotten straight A's since fifth grade, and I hoped to continue that streak all the way through graduation. So yes, you could say I easily stressed about some things, especially school and my grades. However, I was very interested in why stress level came up, and where exactly the nurse was going with this.

"Have you ever noticed, when you're stressed, that you might grab a small part of your hair, and twirl it? Or pull it out?" I was in shock. Wait, these doctors seriously thought I was the one pulling my own hair out? When I got stressed? I wasn't angry, just more caught off guard because I had known from the very beginning that my hair was literally falling out, all by itself. In the shower, when I brushed it, when I straightened it, wherever I was or whatever I was doing, my hair was falling out when it wanted to. I never touched it.

"No, never." I finally answered her, "I know that I'm not pulling my hair out." My response came off pretty straight-forward, so the woman stopped asking questions and moved on.

"Well, it looks like we have everything checked in and up to date; Dr. S will be in with you shortly." The nurse briefly smiled and walked out. I looked over at my mom to see her reaction to all of the questioning. She was calm where she sat.

"Mom, you know I'm not pulling out my hair right?"

"Oh of course not, sweetie, I understand. I know it's been falling out in the shower. I know." There she went again, always catching me when I was about to fall.

After a while of my mom and I chit chatting, there was a quiet knock at the door. It then suddenly opened and Dr. S burst in. She was tall and lean, and strong for her frame. She had dark brown hair, almost appearing black to me, tiny dark brown eyes that were somewhat magnified by her chic glasses, healthy skin, obviously, and a big warm smile. She looked straight at me, hurried over to the bed, and shook my hand excitedly.

"Hi Lesley, I'm Dr. S. Let me take a look here." I tried to process her fast entrance, but then quickly flipped my hair again for her to see. She said some medical terms under her breath that only I could really hear because she was standing so close to me. She fiddled through the rest of my hair, checking for any other spots that were hiding from me. She gently tapped me on the back, and I took that as my cue to sit up all the way.

"Well, Lesley, it definitely looks to me like Alopecia Areata. Now let me explain a bit further about what that really is. Alopecia is a very rare and poorly researched disease. It's an autoimmune disorder. It's not harmful or life threatening to the body, but it's very unpredictable. It generally comes in cycles where you'll lose hair, it'll grow back, and you'll lose it again. Alopecia overall means hair loss…Areata means that the hair loss is in small areas all over the head. Totalis means the hair loss is basically over the entire head, and you lose your hair completely." I could tell she made sure to keep eye contact with me, because I was the patient in the room, and I was the one who needed to understand my own disease. I appreciated her respecting me that way.

Dr. S did her best to explain the disease at my level of comprehension. "Now, what really happens is this. Lesley, your white blood cells, which are the ones that attack bad things in your body like cancer or bacteria…they, for some reason that doctors still don't understand, attack your hair follicles, interpreting them as something harmful. And when they attack your hair, that's what causes your hair to simply fall out in patches. Unfortunately, there's no cure for Alopecia…just some treatments that doctors have tried for patients." I got the concept of what, but still didn't get why. But neither did she, or any doctor, really, for that matter. That's what frustrated me the most.

"Why the heck would my white blood cells just randomly attack my hair? Why? That's not fair," I thought to myself.

Dr. S continued to smile at both my mom and me. She began to discuss with us some treatments and medications she had used with other patients going through similar experiences like mine. She talked about some pills that had the side effect of hair growth, which is what we actually wanted, but she said we'd most likely use those a little further down the road. For that particular day, Dr. S asked if I'd be willing to try Cortisone injections where my two bald spots were. I thought about it for a minute, that Aunt Leslie did it and it worked for her, so it'd work for me, right? And, I mean, I've been getting shots for allergies and what not since I was a baby, so I was used to needles. I talked myself into it and agreed to the shots. Dr. S left the room to gather her necessary materials for the injections.

"Okay Lesley, you ready?" Dr. S kindly asked, after returning and preparing each shot. "Here we go…" I had my iPod earphones in, ready to distract me from the pain. The first prick startled me. I jumped a little, but not enough to throw Dr. S off course. It felt like a bee sting, the needle injecting some kind of poison into my head. The poison would slowly seep into my scalp, eventually spreading out around the actual injected area. She'd quickly move on, and do about fifteen shots for each spot. After every prick, I'd hope that that was the last one, until I felt another one right next to it, stinging my whole scalp again. It felt like every time, she was hitting a nerve or something; I got the chills, start-ing from my head, and then traveling down my spine. I hated every second of it. I glanced down at my iPod, trying to figure out the song title because I wasn't even able to process what song it was. "Please don't cry Les-ley, not now. You're almost done," I repeated over and over again in my mind. I continued staring at the small, pink device until a big, wet tear dropped directly on the screen.

The appointment was finally over. I had slowly walked out of the office, holding down small strips of gauze on the injected areas. They only bled for a short period of time, but my head throbbed like no other. It was such a crazy sensation; my whole scalp felt numb, but at the same time stung with pain. My mom led me out to where we had parked, and opened the door for me. We got into the car, and my mom asked, "You okay, hon?"

"Yeah, I'm fine. I think I'll take a nap on the way back home." She nodded in agreement and started the car. A sudden wave of fatigue rushed through my body. I didn't want to move a muscle. The throbbing contin-ued in my head, and traveled all around. The pulsating rhythm actually put me to sleep. I remember being in that state of "half asleep half awake," when the sun hit my eyes. I kept them closed, but I felt the warm light on my face. Suddenly, the sun was mysteriously cov-ered, and shade returned to my eyes. Confused, I slowly blinked to regain vision, and saw my mom's hand in front of the sun. One hand was on the wheel, the other protecting my tired face from the glare. I was amazed.

"You're a good mommy," I quietly said, as I drifted back to sleep.

Army Attack at Lunch

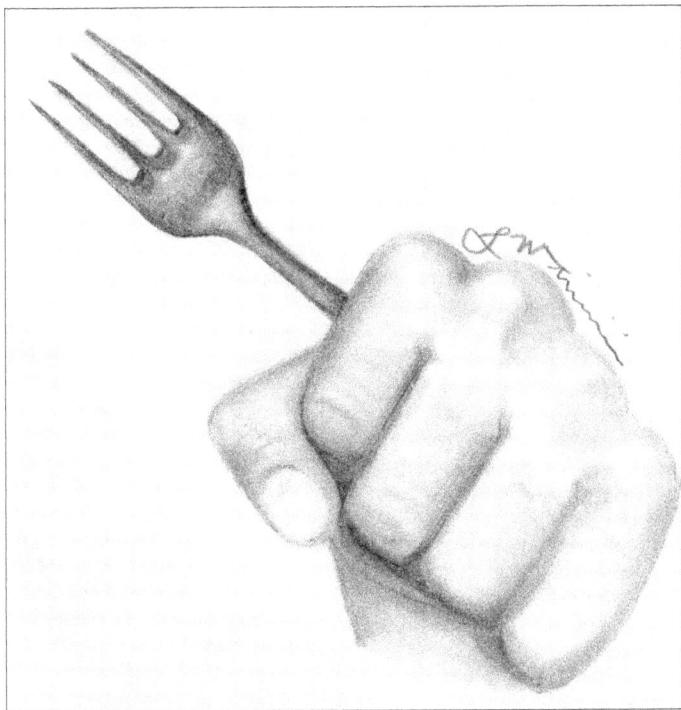

"I'm so glad that you took this disease as a blessing in disguise. You had a decision to make, you could own it, or let it bring you down. You have really grown and prospered from this experience that takes such immense strength and confidence."

~Madi F.

I finished seventh grade, struggling to keep my hair disease a secret from the general population of Deer Creek middle school. Yes, my close friends knew about it, but I didn't really want anyone else to know. Middle school years were already tough with all the puberty changes, the distinct group of friends, and the need to fit in. The overall goal was to be the most popular in those years. Everything seemed to matter: your clothes, your shoes, your weight, your friends, your grades, your personality, and of course, your hair. The pressure to be like everyone else, yet stand out, was constantly on. And the competition grew more intense every single day. The continuous comparisons between one another caused you to meet some of the best friends of your life, and the worst. I thankfully had Catherine by my side through middle school, as well as Madi Fisher and Emily Cooper: some other neighborhood friends that I had known forever.

Then, of course, there was the dating. You probably changed your mind about who you liked once a week, you'd blush every time you saw them, and you most likely sat next to him or her in at least one class. And when you finally worked up the nerve to confess your feelings for that one person, you definitely didn't have the guts to tell them yourself, you had to make sure one of your best friends was willing to do the job for you. You've probably had about one decent conversation with the person, or maybe not even because you just admire them without even talking to them. The person you liked was usually informed a week early about the exact day that you were going to "ask them out." So they did their best to prepare their perfect answer for you.

Once eighth grade came around, I already had my new crush for most of the year, Marc Axcell. In first and second grade, at Bradford Primary, Marc had been a good friend of mine. Then he moved, and not just out of state, but out of the country. He was born in South Africa, moved to Colorado, moved to England in second grade, and then moved back to Colorado in eighth grade. I had never really forgotten about him, he was just placed far back in my mind. I remember hearing he was moving back, and I had never been more excited. I immediately found him on "MySpace", and emailed him just to see if he even recognized me. Of course he did, and we were able to converse a bit before he actually arrived in Colorado, and registered at Deer Creek for school.

It was finally the first day of eighth grade, and I was strolling into school with a few of my friends when I noticed someone familiar standing in the office. I could see his profile through the window to the office; it was Marc. He was in there with his mom, whom I also recognized. Completely ignoring what my friends were saying, I sprinted into the office and excitedly tapped Marc on the back.

"Hi!" I said, with the biggest smile on my face. Both he and his mom quickly turned around.

"Hey! How are you?" He replied. His British accent made me blush, because I hadn't heard him talk like that before.

"I'm good! And you?" I finally said.

"I'm great," he smiled.

"Well it was so good to see you, come find me when you can!" I skipped away, happier than ever. I was so glad to have him there. I knew we'd be close again.

My Alopecia hadn't gotten much worse or better since seventh grade. I still had a couple spots, mainly on the back of my head. My hair was much thinner too. I could tell, and I knew other people could tell also. Fortunately, I was much more open in eighth grade to talk about my disease. I was still super self-conscious and disappointed about it, but I was attempting to live my life with it.

All of the people that knew about my issues had been more than understanding. They were all so respectful and thoughtful towards me. I wasn't asking for sympathy whatsoever, I just hoped for support, and that's exactly what I got from my fellow peers. I found it interesting how each one of them would react differently. There were those who, once I told them, kindly kept quiet and didn't ask one more thing about it. And then there were those who couldn't stop asking questions because they were so interested in the whole disease. I guess I was fine with either reaction; I didn't really care by that point.

Since I opened up more to telling everyone about Alopecia Areata and what I was experiencing because of it, I felt more comfortable in my own skin. Both my family and friends supported me 100 percent, and I couldn't be more thankful. I was finally, but very slowly, getting back on my feet and back into my normal, everyday life. My confidence was coming back in tiny pieces, and overall I started to feel like I'd be okay for the most part. Everyone still accepted me for who I was, right?

After a few months into the school routine at

Deer Creek, lunchtime was what saved all the students from going crazy. We all needed our time to social- ize, eat, and do something active at recess. I remember I was having a good day; nothing dramatic with the friends had happened yet, I had a cute new outfit on, and my hair was down. As I rushed down the stairs in a pack of starving students, I smiled to myself. I was okay, I was happy, and I was about to see all of my amazing friends and spend the next 45 minutes with them.

I entered the large opening to the cafeteria, and searched for my friends. I looked around, observing all of the tables with friends that devoured food, or ones that couldn't stop laughing about some inside joke. I knew where my friends would generally be sitting because all of the cliques in middle school owned and defended where they sat everyday. A specific table seemed to be the actual "property" of one group; I thought it was ridiculous. After a while of standing at the front of the cafeteria, I spotted Marc and Madi at the end of a table with a bunch of other friends. Just as I began to make my way over there with a huge grin on my face, something suddenly stopped me.

"Hey, you know you have a bald spot on the back of your head," said a voice from close behind me. I remember freezing up like I had just been stabbed with the sharpest words ever, and I couldn't move. My smile vanished and my face grew tense. A feeling of heat then flushed through my body and I barely felt sweat forming on my forehead. I was stunned out of embar- rassment. I turned around, trying to anticipate who the person was. It was a short, heavy kid from my last class; I didn't even know his name. He was known for his rudeness with teachers and other people.

"What?" I said harshly. I wasn't literally asking the question of "what," like I didn't hear what he had said. I asked it in a way of saying "why on earth would you say something like that?" Instead, he took it as the literal way.

"I said, you have a bald spot on the back of your head, like right there," he repeated. He lifted his finger to a spot on the back of his head, trying to show me exactly where it was located. Of course I knew where it was. Of course I knew I had a bald spot, more than one actually. I did not need someone to personally point it out to me. Did he seriously think I had no idea about it? Was he expecting me to jump up, gasp in amazement, and say, "Omigosh, thank you I had no clue that was there!" I was in pure shock. I didn't respond, and continued to stare at him. My eyes filled with tears and I felt like I was going to explode. I could see he was growing uncomfortable with the way I was looking at him. I swiftly turned and dashed towards Marc and my friends. I stumbled over to where Marc sat on the corner of the bench, and pushed him over so there was room for me to sit. I tried telling him exactly what happened, but instead, buried my face in my hands. I was a mess, and I couldn't even grasp what that kid had said to me.

"Lesley, what the heck happened?! What's wrong?!" Marc grabbed my shoulders, trying to turn me around so he could see me. I lifted my head and continued to cry so hard that I couldn't even get a word out. I knew other people had noticed the dramatic scene I was causing, but I didn't care one little bit. They were all a blur to me.

"Les, calm down. Calm down, it's okay, what happened?" He asked again. By this time, I had drawn all of the attention at the table. Everyone looked at me, waiting anxiously for an answer. I focused on Marc, slowed my breathing down, and slowly caught my breath.

"That kid, over there, he said…well I was walking over to you and he was behind me and he said like, 'you know there's a bald spot on the back of your head.'" I broke down again and turned away from the rest of the listeners. Marc knew exactly who had said it. He got up, and so did half of the table. Madi and Emily quickly came over to comfort me. I watched Marc walk over to the kid and get straight up in his face, explaining to him exactly what he had just done.

After a couple minutes, Marc finished, and a pack of girls took his place. It seemed as if the whole cafeteria had heard what the kid had said, and one by one, they wanted to tell him off. Through my blurry vision, I watched in amazement, girls I had never talked to in my entire life got up and yelled something at him because they were so furious. It looked like a swarm of bees were invading him.

I especially remember one of my other good friends, Jordan Davidson, getting up to talk to him. I met her in my seventh grade Spanish class. She was a total sweetheart, and we became close friends almost immediately. Out of all of my friends, she by far, grew the most protective over me with my Alopecia. I had never seen her more upset than on this day. She later told me how frustrated she was that someone couldn't use simple common sense. That even though he didn't know the situation or that I had a disease, he should have thought, just a little, before he blurted out something like that.

As I watched kid after kid get in his face, I suddenly felt bad for him; I had a complete army attacking him because of the one thing he said. Of course that wasn't my intention—to make him feel so ashamed about what he did. But apparently, I just had a lot of protective friends sticking up for me, and I don't think he was prepared for them at all. I had sympathy for him, though, in a bigger picture. I knew he was insecure with himself because of other things that didn't even relate to this. We all were.

I had finally stopped crying, and then began trying to calm the others down, or at least the ones I knew. Once everyone backed off a bit, the kid was visible again. He looked beyond overwhelmed, turned around, and walked away. I took a deep breath, and walked outside with my friends to recess. He and I never talked after that day. He never apologized to me, and I never had anything more to say to him.

After thinking about it, I came to the realization that in junior high, every single student is so sensitive, fragile, and simply broken. We have all shattered into bits and pieces, and we have no idea where or how to start picking them up, and putting them back together. We take everything someone says or does personally. We don't even think for a second that maybe they were referring to someone else, or that they didn't mean what they really said.

Everyone wants to vent their own anxiety, and the cafeteria scene was the perfect opportunity for them to do so. That's why people I had never even talked to before got up, and voiced their opinion. It's because they finally got their chance to say something to someone who had pointed out a flaw. We all had our problems and this was the first time someone had the guts to point one out. And just look how we all reacted, because it hit home for every individual. I was still facing the world with my flaws in public view, and because of that honesty, everyone in the room felt their human vulnerabilities exposed. Even though it happened to just me, everyone could relate to it.

Maybe we could all learn from this, and start to watch what we say more carefully. Take an extra moment to think how your words will affect the person you're addressing. Try putting yourself in their position; did they fail an important test last class? Were they in a fight with a friend? Were they having a good day? Respect that everybody has vulnerabilities, and you have the power to lift them up or knock them down with what you say and how you say it. Maybe if that kid had commented to me in a better way, things might have gone differently.

Never Trust a Hat

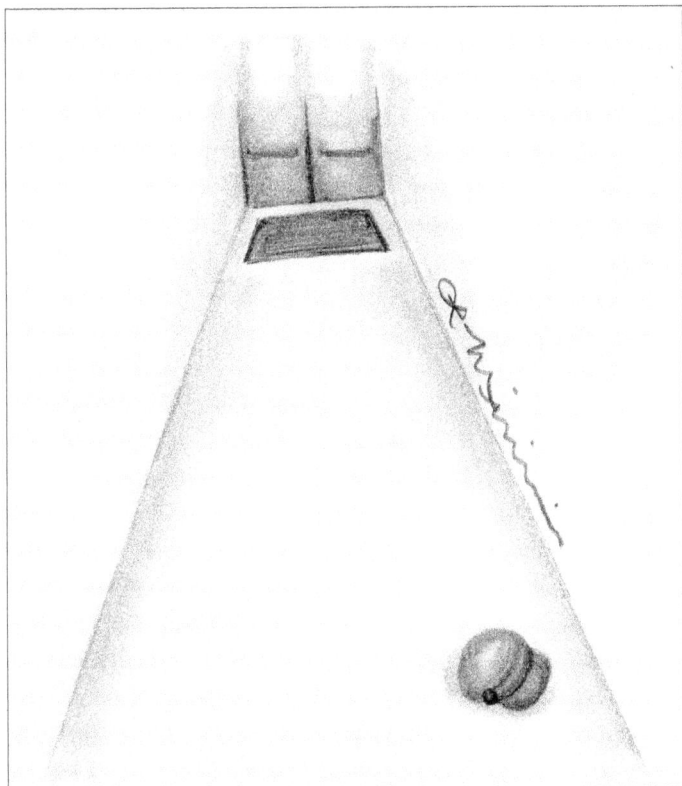

"I just want to tell you that I admire you for always being so happy with all you've been through with your hair and everything…I'm just impressed."

~Jensen T.

I could not wait to be in high school. Chatfield Senior High was only about five minutes away, and I remember pointing it out whenever we drove by, and just imagining what it'd be like when I went there. My class got lucky, because the year we came was right after they decided to re-do the entire entrance, extend the parking lot, put in soccer fields and tennis courts, and build a complete additional wing. It was like walking into a brand new school as freshmen; we all loved it. I was going to be with all of my good friends, plus my brother.

I would be arriving as a freshman, and my brother, Michael, would be a senior that same year. He and I hadn't been at the same school since I was in kindergarten and he was in third grade at Bradford Primary. We were two and a half years apart in age, but three years in school. Michael and I became extremely close during our high school years.

However, when the two of us were much younger, he always found me an easy target to pick on, annoy, and physically hurt whenever he felt like it was necessary. It seemed like all of our home videos with Michael and me as toddlers always ended with my dad repeatedly yelling "Michael" and having to suddenly turn off the camera in order to stop Michael and save me. You could say we were just like any other ordinary siblings, but it was probably a bit more intense than that. I was a fragile toy to Michael, but he rarely took that into consideration, so I was forced to grow more resistant to him.

For some odd reason, I completely admired him. He'd knock me down; I'd pout for a bit, but then get right back up. I wanted to be like him, or at least as strong as him, so I tried not to be so weak around him. Of course

I'd get upset when he never listened to me, or when he just randomly tackled me, or when he decided that giving me a dead arm (you know, the torturous action of incessantly pounding the same spot over and over until the muscle feels dead) was the best solution to whatever our pathetic argument was about. But, I knew that he'd come around eventually. I knew that even though some referred to him as the "devil child," he'd be fine in the end; I just didn't know when his transformation would take place.

I believe that everything happens for a reason. As you already know, I regularly attended church. Now that I was older and more mature, my relationship with God was becoming more personal. Instead of Sunday Mass being the only time I set aside for truly thinking about who God is, what He means to me, how He works in the world, and specifically in the life of a freshman in high school, now I was preparing for Confirmation. For those of you who aren't Catholic, let me explain… Confirmation is a special occasion, which marks a recognition of a deeper understanding of one's personal faith and growing walk with Christ. In my studies, I was learning that God had some sort of life plan just for me, which gave me the confidence to believe that nothing happens by mistake.

God knew I needed someone to be able to push me around, and then completely ignore me when all I wanted was attention. That little mind game caused me to mentally and emotionally grow stronger because I'd only have myself to look to at that point. I also grew that much more independent because of Michael. As much as he'd physically hurt me, God knew the whole time that, in the long run, he was empowering me. And now

I know for sure that God gave me Michael as a brother in order to help me develop the strength of character to handle my future challenges.

Things finally changed between us, close to when Michael himself was a freshman. He was put in a different environment with new friends, new classes, new problems, and new excitements. And that's exactly what he needed in order to reveal his hidden sweet side. All of a sudden, instead of punching me when he walked by, he'd hug me. Instead of me constantly flinching when he made a slight movement, I'd stay calm because I knew he wouldn't hurt me anymore. It was one of the best changes in my life, and his too. Michael and I grew closer and closer as brother and sister from that time on.

Starting school at Chatfield, I surprisingly had a full head of hair. I had some bald spots the year before, but because of the injections and other medications I was on, the summertime gave my hair the opportunity to start growing back. Even with most of my hair, I wasn't sure how the new high school crowd would react to the situation. The majority of Deer Creek middle school students knew about my Alopecia, but now there were at least three other schools that funneled into Chatfield, and none of them had a clue. I was hoping because my hair started to grow back at the beginning of the year, so would my confidence. And I hoped I could almost forget about it altogether. I didn't want this disease to be one more thing to worry about as I entered high school. I have to admit though, I was afraid it was too good to be true.

As the end of the first semester approached, I started going through another cycle of hair loss. The spots were still disguisable for the most part, but I had a feeling the hair loss wasn't going to stop this time around. As my hair continued to fall out in patches, I really began to notice how thin my hair appeared. It was the complete opposite of what I was used to: having full, thick, black hair. By this point, I couldn't cover up the spots with certain hairstyles anymore. I had to find another solution.

My close friends knew how bad my hair loss was getting, so I told them about my plan of wearing hats. My mom helped me pick out a couple of cute ones, and then my friends jumped in also. For instance, Sarah Dubetz, another grade school/neighborhood friend, had always been super caring for others, and me, especially because of my Alopecia. She came to school that week with a gift, and gave it to me in class. I was shocked, because I had no idea what it was and what it was for. I did my best to open it secretly, without disturbing the rest of the students. I carefully and quietly unwrapped the tissue paper in the box; it was a hat. By far, the cutest one I had, too. It was mainly blue, with a plaid design, and a brown bow on the side of it. After admiring it, I looked up at Sarah, completely speechless. She just smiled back, and asked if I liked it. I absolutely loved it, and I couldn't stop thanking her. It was little things like that that truly showed how thoughtful people could be.

*   *   *

Chatfield has off periods and off campus lunches, and because Michael was allowed to drive then, friends and I kindly took advantage of him. He didn't mind, just because he was always going out to eat somewhere, now he got to take a few extra people. He and I got along for the most part, and all of my friends seemed to love Michael because of his playful and entertaining personality.

For the first semester of freshmen year, our "clan" consisted of Marc Axcell, Jensen Teague, Erica Smith, my brother, and me. I had known Jensen since grade school, just like Marc. He was by far one of the sweetest kids I knew, so I loved to be around him. When Marc moved back from England, he and Jensen hit it off well.

I met Erica in fourth grade; we had both tried out for Rush league competitive soccer. That year, our recreational teams were splitting up, so moving on to a competitive league was the next step. We were both put on the A-one team. All of the girls were new to each other, but Erica stood out to me right from the beginning. For a while, the whole team was quiet, but as individuals began speaking up, I could tell how funny Erica was. We made each other laugh uncontrollably during practices, and quickly became best friends. She lived close; however, she went to a small private Catholic school. So we weren't able to see each other much, except for at soccer. Right before high school, she quit soccer altogether so she could focus on basketball, family, and other things, so we almost never saw each other. But fortunately, because she lived close, and because her older sister was going to Chatfield in my brother's grade, her parents agreed for her to go there also. I could not wait to spend high school with her!

The five of us spent lunch together basically every day. We would all meet up right in front of the bridge to the front doors, and then usually try to agree on a place to eat. It became a sort of ritual between all of us; we all knew where to be, what time, where Michael parked, etc… But I remember one day perfectly in particular. It was during the time my hair was falling out fast, and I wore my variety of hats for about a week. I knew people would be wondering why I suddenly began wearing hats all the time, but I couldn't worry too much about that. It had become my last resort until I could figure out my next disguise.

That day, I was wearing a really cute dark green "chapeau." The remaining hair I had was bundled in a small ponytail, which was then tucked up into the back of my hat. It was lunchtime, so I found Erica first and then walked with her to the bridge. Michael, Jensen, and Marc were waiting for us right there. I could already tell the boys were in one of their moods. As much as I loved these three musketeers, they could occasionally get out of control because they fed off of each other. If one teased me, the other two jumped in on it. Erica would do her best to defend me, but it was hard with them. Even though they joked around a lot, almost always, I'll admit I took it too personally.

They had already decided to go to McDonalds. Erica and I weren't exactly in the mood for that lunch choice, so of course I voiced my opinion.

"Uh yeah, Michael we don't really wanna go there. Sorry."

"Well guess what. We are. We're going there so deal with it," he jokingly replied.

"No, Michael. Not today." I said sternly.

For just a split second, the young Michael took over, the one where he didn't think whatsoever before he acted. This was when he would do something, and not consider the consequences. He suddenly snatched my hat, and chucked it! (You may insert appropriate expletive here.) He had just thrown my comfort zone down the bridge hallway. I couldn't believe it. I kept trying to rewind it, but I knew I couldn't when I saw my green hat, disfigured on the ground about ten feet from me. Everyone that passed was staring, including Marc and Jensen, so I ran to my hat, picked it up and threw it back on my head. Then, I rushed down to the commons, hoping to find somewhere to hide for the moment. Erica was right behind me, struggling to keep up. She and I ran down the stairs and around the corner of a wall. I didn't even glance back in the boys' direction.

"Erica, I can't believe he would do that! I mean… you saw that. He literally threw my hat across the hall!"

"I know, I know, Les. I can't even believe it either. But it's okay, it's over with now." Erica did her best to calm me down, but I was furious. I was so embarrassed too, because it was my own brother who did it. My geography teacher was walking by, when she saw me freaking out. She hurried over to me, asking what had happened. I tried to explain to her the situation, but the hall was too loud, and I was too flustered. Before I could even get a complete sentence out, she reached out and held me so close to her I was afraid of getting tears on her pretty blouse. But she didn't care one bit, she just continued to hug me and tell me it was okay now. She held me like I was her own daughter, she was being my mother figure at the time, and I calmed down in a matter of minutes.

She finally let me pull back and I slowly looked up at her. She had the most concerned look on her face; I thought she might cry too. She recognized Erica was there for me, and would now take over. She gave me one last quick hug and rushed back to whatever she was off to do before she spotted me. Erica rubbed my back until I caught my breath. She was right there for me the entire time, and had no intention of leaving. Erica and I decided to find a place to sit, and spend the rest of lunch there, at school. We tried talking about it, but both didn't want to get worked up again, so we found other topics to distract us.

The bell rang for class to start. Neither of us got up right away, and she continued to look at me, checking to make sure I was okay. I picked up my big bag of books and supplies, swung it around my shoulder, and gave her a big hug. As I began walking to geometry, someone grabbed my arm. I turned around to see Marc.

"Lesley…he feels really bad. He didn't mean to. It was just him not thinking before he did it. He's really sorry, and I know he'll talk to you later about it. But I thought I'd tell you, he feels bad."

"Okay." I simply said, and walked away. I couldn't figure out exactly what I was feeling. I wanted to forgive him, I mean, he was my brother who I saw every single day. But I was still so angry inside, and I needed more time to think about it. I walked into geometry class and found my seat without saying hi to any of my friends. I swung my book bag down to the floor, and was about to dig for my calculator, when I saw a small paper bag on top of everything. I opened the bag up, and it was two chocolate chip cookies from McDonalds. "Marc must have snuck them in there when I was walking away," I thought. They were pretty cold and stale. I got up, walked to the corner of the room where the trash can was, and threw them away. I wasn't ready to forgive Michael, not yet.

Later that day after school, when I had calmed

down, Michael and I talked for a while. I could tell he was sincerely sorry, and that he didn't understand what he was doing at that specific moment. He was my brother, my crazy but caring brother who I loved, and I quickly accepted his apology.

As I thought about it, the situation with Michael is a perfect example of someone not thinking before they act. Just like in junior high, when that boy said something to me without even really contemplating what he said, how it would affect me, or how it would affect others. Michael was obviously not intentionally trying to hurt me, but he did. And it was all because of one small action that blew up out of proportion. It happened because he wasn't thinking or looking ahead to what the consequences may be. He simply acted in a completely different state of mind; frustrated because I was argumentative when they had already chosen a lunch place. Once again, it became obvious how important it is to acknowledge your own reactions to certain dilemmas, because they are always capable of harming other individuals. If only Mickey D's had sounded appetizing that day...

I Finally Have Barbie™ Hair

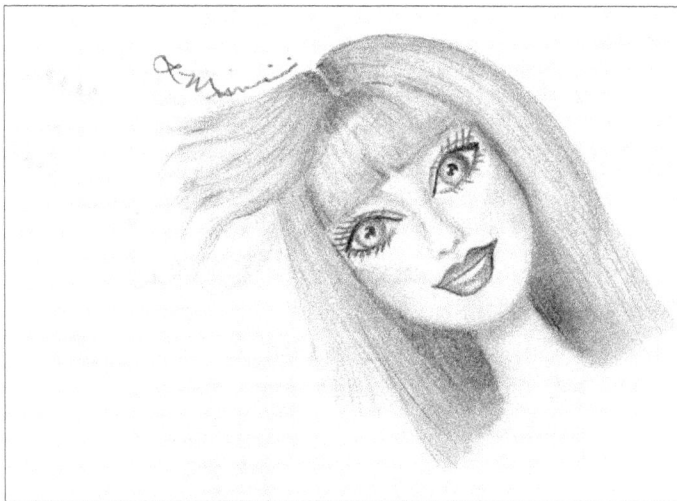

"I admire you and your strength. It really made me think twice about how much I complain about having diabetes when there is no reason to after hearing your story. And to be honest, I always thought that was your real hair anyway!"

~Erin B.

My one-week of wearing hats wasn't going to miraculously make everything better like I hoped for. My hats were the next thing I turned to for a feeling of comfort, but that was quickly pulled away from me after experiencing how delicate they were themselves: a.k.a. easily removable and thrown. My remaining hair, my scalp, and my self-esteem was already too fragile, so I needed something stronger that would overpower all of those insecurities. Nothing I thought of, though, seemed to be powerful enough to make me feel confident again.

I continued to lose more and more hair in the shower. Small patches would secretly fall out, almost as if they were sneaking off my head and down the drain where I couldn't see them. I tried not to look down much; I knew I couldn't handle it. Because of the amount of hair I was losing, the water I used for showering would sit around in the bathtub because the drain was so clogged up. Even if I were in the shower for about fifteen minutes, I'd have water up to my shins because it couldn't go down. Finally, when the water found a chance to seep through the drain, the hair I had lost during that shower was totally visible and exposed, all tangled up and scattered around the tub.

Fortunately, I have a father that would do literally anything for me. I haven't told you much about Dad until now. His support is so constant, it's easy to forget just how much he gives all the time. He never asks for recognition although he deserves it. For example, every morning, after I showered, got ready, and went to school with my brother, my dad would come upstairs, completely unclog the drain, and clean out all of the hair. He knew I couldn't see that, at least not then. He did his best to make it seem like normal, and like it had never happened.

The clogged drain was like all of my emotions. I would let all that sadness and frustration build up inside of me while I was in the shower, just like the water would get higher and higher. I'd get out in a hurry, knowing that I was about to burst and let everything fall through, but I never did, just like the drain. And then as the day went on, I'd slowly let all of that emotion disappear and get cleaned up, just like my dad did to the bathtub. I definitely couldn't have gotten through that stage without him.

However, that one shower I can remember like it was just yesterday. It was on a Saturday morning, and all of my family was gone. My parents were working out or running errands, and who knows where my brother was. I had slept in like I usually did on the weekends, because it was the only way I could truly catch up on sleeping hours from the previous school week. I was dreading the idea of taking a shower, but I knew I had to because the thin straggly hair that remained on my head appeared way too greasy and I couldn't stand that.

I rubbed my eyes multiple times in order to wake myself up. I sat up and waited for a bit, trying to make out every object in my room. It took a while because my room was always extremely dark. My friends called it "the black cave;" because my blinds were so thick and in one piece of fabric, that when they were down over the window, not one speck of light could enter my room. I loved it that way. But when I woke up, there was no way I could tell what time it was—it was that dark. I glanced at my phone, ignoring the couple of new text messages I had, and in the corner I saw 10: something. "Whatever,"

I thought. Not too early, not too late. I had plans to go out with some friends that evening, like see a movie or something. So I decided to shower first thing.

I turned on the water, adjusted it to my favorite temperature, and stepped in. I had a weird feeling about that day, something wasn't right, but I shook it off. I knew I'd lose some more hair probably but come on, showers don't last forever, right?

I cautiously raised my hands to my head, anticipating what exactly would happen when I massaged the conditioner through my hair. In a matter of seconds, as I glimpsed down at my trembling hands, I noticed two handfuls of hair that had completely fallen out. I collapsed onto the frigid bathtub surface, hysterically crying in dismay. Everything merged into a colossal blur. The water from the showerhead above me, and my tears mingled together, making it impossible to see, and impossible for me to wrap my head around the fact that I was losing my hair…all of it.

I lay down in the tub, curled up in an awkward position and cried. I cried my eyes out. I cried loud enough that I knew someone would hear me eventually, except that my family was gone…I felt so alone in my own house, and thoroughly isolated from everyone I knew. "No one has this," I thought, "No one is going through this like I am." I cried crazy hard. You know the kind, the one where there's not any air left to gasp in and then suddenly you scream out again. Without noticing, I leaned back slowly, into the path of the water. The water poured down into my mouth, causing me to cough and snap out of the dramatic scene I was making for myself. At this point I sat up, which for some reason, took all of the energy I had left in me at the moment. I just felt so weak and full of despair. I finally turned the water off. To this day, I have no idea how long I was in the bathtub that morning. It could have been five minutes, or even thirty minutes, all I know was that the water was getting colder by the minute.

I stood up, grabbed my towel and buried my face in it. There was no way I was going to look in the mirror then. I didn't want to see what difference that insane amount of hair loss did. I didn't know anything yet; did I still have hair? Was it completely gone now? I was not ready to see what had happened, so I avoided the mirror.

I wrapped the towel around me, ran to my room and snatched some comfy clothes that were on the floor. I knew I'd have to review the damage at some point, so I did my best to prepare myself. I held my breath and stepped in front of my closet mirror. First I noticed how red my face was from crying. I could barely see my eyes because of the puffiness, and my nose was running. This definitely didn't help me feel any prettier. Finally, I looked at my hair…there was still some, but barely any. I was actually somewhat surprised at how much had stayed, but it had certainly taken a beating that shower. I lifted up some strands of hair, examining the areas that were bald. So much was gone now, and I had no clue how I'd be able to disguise it. It looked ridiculous to me, and I threw my hands down in frustration. I stomped over to the phone, dialed my mom's cell phone number and waited anxiously for her voice.

"Hello?" She answered.

"Mom it's gone. My hair is gone; all of it fell out in the shower. Well not all, but so much of it, Mom it's crazy! Like half of it! No, no, more than half! I won't even look in the mirror, it's not me. I hate this so much!"

"Lesley, Lesley, please! Sweetheart, omigosh I am so sorry…please just calm down…we're going to figure this out, I promise. It's okay, I'll be home very soon and I'll check it out. You know, I know you're not crazy about this idea Les, but I really think we need to consider a wig possibly. Just think about it…okay don't you worry, I'm almost home. I love you."

"Love you too, bye," I quietly said, keeping myself from crying again. As a freshman in high school, I hated the thought of wearing a wig. Hair was still such a big deal to girls, and the last thing I wanted mine to be was fake. The only wig I had really seen was my mom's when she went through chemotherapy and breast cancer. And that wig, no offense to her, looked extremely phony. Plus, I also thought a wig would just fly away in the wind or fall off if someone tugged on it. I didn't want to experience that kind of embarrassment, and I didn't want that paranoid feeling back again. I didn't want to have to explain to all of my friends at school why I suddenly had thick, healthy, long, black hair compared to the scraggly strands they saw yesterday. All of this stuff I didn't want, but what I truly needed was comfort and happiness again. I needed a wig no matter what I kept telling myself.

I cancelled my plans that night. I wasn't ready to go out and show everyone I had lost half of my hair. Instead, I spent the evening evaluating my situation. I had run out of silly ideas to disguise my patchy scalp. No more specific hairstyles, no more strategic black eye shadow on the translucent bald spots, no more hats. I had also run out of hope. I asked myself why God would choose me to deal with this. Apparently God had more faith in me than I ever thought I'd have in myself. The more I thought about it all, the more I came to the conclusion that I could not give up, not just yet. Maybe a wig wouldn't be so bad after all; I had to at least try it, right?

The next day, after my mom had thoroughly searched for some of the best wig places in town, she narrowed it down to two. One was in downtown Littleton, and the other was in Cherry Creek. I had no special preference, so we decided to try the Cherry Creek one. Of course, I took Catherine along because I needed my support and some "girl to girl" opinion. And then both of my parents came as well. We planned on going to church right after, so it was easier to all be together.

I remember parking on the side of a road, going down some stairs and then circling around a wall that put us right in front of the wig shop. Catherine and I rushed in first, and suddenly stopped when a room full of various wigs surrounded us. There were so many different colors, styles, and lengths! Each wig was placed on a mannequin's head, lined up next to one another. I couldn't believe it. A wave of excitement hit me, and all I wanted to do was start trying some on.

A young, pretty Asian woman calmly approached all of us and introduced herself. She told us to look around, and pick out some that we thought might work. Then she would assist putting them on me, and possibly trim up or thin out any bulk in the wig. She also mentioned how there are two main types of wig hair: synthetic and real. Real hair was way out of our budget range at the time, so we stuck with synthetic.

The only time I had heard of synthetic hair was with my good old Barbie™ Dolls. I remember one of

my favorite Barbie™ girls in particular, with the traditional blonde, long, straight hair. And for some reason,
I so badly wanted her to have curly hair. My mom had
curled my hair a lot as a child, so I thought, "Hey, why
not try it on Barbie™?" After minutes of constant asking
and pouting to my mother, she finally said "yes", even
though she warned me about how Barbie's™ hair isn't
meant to be curled, it's not like real hair. But I couldn't
tell the difference, so I was determined to try it. One
touch of the steaming curling iron and a chunk of Barbie's™ perfect hair sizzled right off. I was devastated, but
soon remembered what my mom had said, so I couldn't
blame her. That's all I really knew about synthetic hair
at that point.

I knew I wanted my wig to look very similar to my
regular hair color and style. Catherine and I spotted a
couple, but one stood out to both of us. It was jet black,
straight, long and shiny. It looked like me. We pointed
that one out and the woman walked over, took it off the
mannequin and brought it to me. She motioned for me
to sit down at a big chair in front of a mirror. I sat down,
not knowing if I was more excited or nervous. I really
needed this to work out; I needed it to look like I imag-
ined it. The hair I had left was already pushed back out
of sight when the wig went on. The woman made a few
adjustments, placing the hairs where she wanted them.
I looked in the mirror and absolutely loved it. It didn't
even look fake! I peered over at Catherine and my parents, all of them in complete awe.

"Do you like it?" I asked, trying not to smile too
big.

"Yes Lesley I love it!" Catherine exclaimed.

"Lesley you look beautiful. It's just like your real

hair." My dad said. My mom nodded and agreed. They all admired it, and so did I. The lady was smiling also, and took our reaction as a "yes, this is the one." She began to take a little bit of the bulk out, and I asked if she could add some layers and side bangs. Before I knew it, the wig was done, and it was mine. I couldn't believe I had fallen for it so fast. It felt like my hair, my own hair again and there were no bald spots to throw me off guard.

After paying, Catherine and I rushed outside to discover it was raining. At first I was scared, I didn't want my new purchase to get wet or ruined. But I knew it'd be okay. The two of us sprinted up the stairs and down the street a little to the car. We unlocked the door and jumped in the back seat. I had the biggest grin across my face as we both tried to catch our breath. I couldn't believe that the wig had stayed on that whole time. I had literally just bolted out of the wig shop without it even budging. Not to mention how it was also pouring rain. I guess once you have the wig on, it just kind of stays on. It ends up fitting to its owner's head perfectly in a matter of days. As simple as it is to personally remove, when it comes to rain, wind, or running, it's a completely different situation. That's when it takes on the shape of your head, and won't fall off. It fascinated me.

"Les, I like it so much. It looks so pretty on you." Catherine said, breathing hard in between her words.

"Thank you." I said, then turned to her and gave her one of the biggest hugs. My parents hustled to the car as well, and got in right after us. Everyone was a little damp, but no one cared. We were off to church now, and that would be the first big public area that I showed myself with my first wig.

We were a bit late to Mass, not knowing exactly how long finding the right wig would take. But it didn't matter because Catherine's family was already there, saving seats for us. Michelle had called my mom earlier to describe where they were sitting, so once we entered, my mom took the lead. It was during a song when we walked in; we found the Arends and quickly squished into the pew. Soon after, the song ended, and everyone in church sat down.

My heart was racing, all of the adrenalin pumping through my blood. Were people staring at me? Could they tell it was a wig? Did they notice how perfect it looked? Suddenly, Catherine nudged me and signaled for me to look down the pew at her mom. I leaned forward, and so did Michelle. She looked at me, gave me a thumbs-up, and mouthed, "I love your hair". I whispered "thank you" back to her, and turned forward once again. I stopped questioning who was looking at me and why. I didn't care anymore. I had beautiful hair now. I was with God, and a room full of holy, joyful people, a room with no judgment.

I finally realized how broken down you need to be before a solution can be presented to you. You need be beaten to the core, hanging on by your last thread. You need to be on the verge of giving up and losing everything, and not know what will happen next. You kind of wait there, at your lowest, just to see who or what will pick you up and put you back on your feet.

God gave me my friends and family. Plus, He helped me find my first wig. That wig was the only thing that would fix my "problem." All I needed to do was trust in it; believe that it would work for me. And it did. And the reason I was able to trust in the wig is because I could trust in God and His plan for me. I mean look, He made sure the next place I went to after getting my wig was His house. He knew the people there would accept me because they were there to worship Him, and focus on Him. They weren't going to judge me, and He knew it was a safe place for me to reveal my new confidence.

Can You Hold This Please?

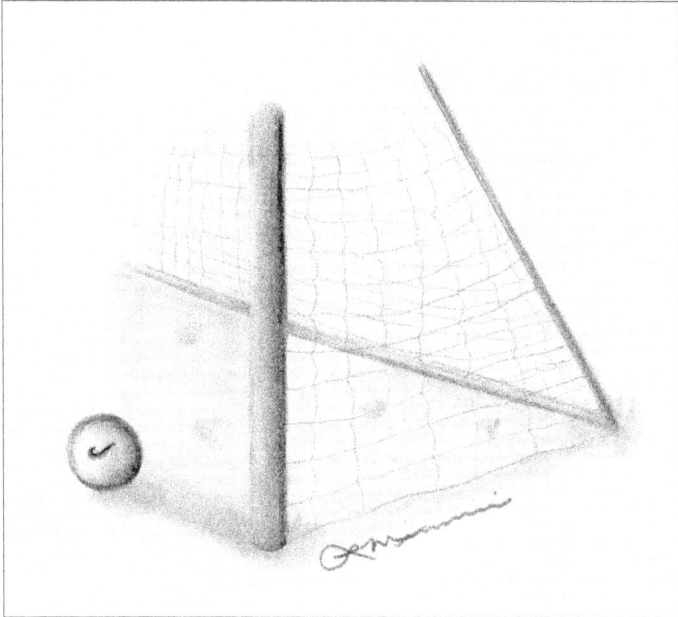

"You always look at the bright side of things, stand up for yourself, and see life's challenges as an event to grow as a person. You are a true inspiration to both me and my family."

~Taylor O.

I've been playing soccer ever since I was five years old. I played for the "Purple Cheetahs," and you could say we thought we were pretty hardcore. Or maybe more realistically, like a bunch of neighborhood girls got together back in Ken Caryl Valley to occasionally kick around a soccer ball. We all somewhat knew each other from living on the same block, seeing each other at the Community Center pool, or even going to school together. Christina and Catherine were both on my team at one point. Catherine lasted for one season; she found other sports and activities more amusing. And Christina played with us all the way up until she found out she was moving to Arizona.

In fourth grade, my recreational team split up, like most did, and we each had the option to move on to a competitive league. About 75 percent of the girls from my team did, and most went to Rush Soccer. That was the most popular league that played within the Littleton location. After a week of tryouts, I was placed on the A-1 (Advanced One); that's basically the third team out of five or six teams in the age group. And I was satisfied there.

There was something about soccer that I loved, more than anything. When I was young, I played tennis, took dance classes, did gymnastics, and much more. But all of those other activities seemed to gradually slip away as I focused more and more on soccer. The funny thing is that I was better at some of the other hobbies than I was at soccer. My mom still remembers how my dance teacher called her immediately after I quit, just to say how talented she thought I was when it came to dancing, and she only hoped I would stay with it. In gymnastics, as a six year old, I was put up with the nine and ten year olds. And in tennis, I had one of my coaches mention to me how I would be a great high school player because of my "lefty spin" and concentration. But soccer was truly what I wanted to do, even though I wasn't the best at it. I had the most fun playing it. Sadly, in high school, girl's tennis and soccer are both spring sports; so I was forced to choose, and I chose soccer.

I had always heard both negative and positive things about high school sports. Negatively, I heard how political, stressful, competitive, and time consuming they were. On the positive side, I heard how much you could improve, how in shape you could get, and close you could get with your entire team. Overall, each side proved to be true for me. But first going into it, I wasn't exactly sure what to expect.

At the beginning of freshman year, I had decided to play soccer in the spring. However, I was not expecting my hair to suddenly fall out in December, so my plans were a bit altered. Playing soccer with a wig on definitely crossed my mind, but I felt like it would be impossible. I mean in soccer, you run, jump, collide, and head the ball. I felt like that was too much for a wig to take on, at least my first one. So I didn't risk it. Instead, I found the solution of wearing a simple "beanie" when I played. I know what you're thinking, I told you to never trust a hat, but this was no pretty decoration, it was a tight fitted hug-my-head elastic beanie.

When I lost my hair in December, Indoor soccer was just about to start up. And the complexes we usually play at are extremely cold because of no heat, so my beanie might come in handy more than I initially thought. I remember when my first game for Indoor came around, I was totally nervous about wearing the hat and what the other girls would think. Thankfully, my team was completely fine with it, acting as if they didn't even notice, or probably just didn't even care. It was still me, still Lesley, and I was the exact same soccer player and teammate to them.

The majority of my team had stayed together throughout the years, so we had all bonded over a large amount of time, which allowed them to see and help me go through the experience I was taking on. But what scared me the most was what the opposing team would think, or the cute, younger referee guys. I stepped onto the turf field, just waiting to get some of the craziest looks. But I didn't. The other team didn't even do a double take, and then I specifically remember how the ref looked at me, smiled, and then asked me, "Ready?" I smiled back and nodded. He blew the whistle, and I played just like any other girl out there with their long ponytails.

The spring season snuck up on me, and I hesitated on playing because of the hair situation. But seriously? I wasn't going to let my appearance of wearing a beanie stop me from playing a sport I loved. As afraid as I was, I decided to play, and went out for tryouts. Unfortunately, the week before, I got very sick and found out I had strep throat. My doctor suggested for me not to play the first two days because I was contagious. This obviously frustrated me and caused me to stress even more; less time of tryouts meant even more pressure. I tried out for the last three days, giving it my all and playing my hardest even though my health wasn't close to its best. I played through the exhaustion and the thought of strangers and upperclassmen looking at me. "Whatever," I thought, "I am here to play soccer, and only that."

Chatfield is known for its outstanding soccer records and achievements. For some reason, Chatfield always got some of the greatest, most talented players in the area. Those girls were the ones that came from the Nike teams—the top teams for the Rush League. I wasn't expecting to make Varsity or even JV freshman year. And that's exactly what happened; I was put on one of the two Level Three teams that were under JV. I was a little upset, considering the circumstances I was playing under, but I quickly got over it.

The second day of training with my new team, I decided I wanted to let all of them know exactly why I would be wearing a beanie, and I only asked for their support and understanding. My good soccer friend, Taylor Ohman, who had played with me on Rush and was now on the Level Three team with me, was the one who had my back the whole time. She pushed for me to get up in front of everyone before practice that day, and say what I needed to. She promised to help or add in anything if I started to have trouble. So I asked my coach if I could quickly speak to the girls about my hair disease before practice, and she kindly agreed. I took a deep breath, got to the front of the classroom that we always met in, and waited anxiously for all the chattering to subside. My coach announced that I had something to share, and the room grew quiet. I still didn't know the girls that well, but I was set on letting them all know.

"Hi. Some of you guys already know me, but I'm Lesley. And I just wanted to say that I'll be wearing a beanie hat like this for the season because I have a hair loss disease called Alopecia...so I don't have all of my hair, and at school I wear a wig, but for soccer, I thought it'd be easier to just wear this. I hope you guys are okay with that, but yeah, I just thought you guys should know…"

"Well that's awesome. We'll have to get you a really cute beanie or something!" a girl that everyone referred to as Spale (that was her last name), blurted out after my speech. A sudden wave of relief rushed over me after hearing Spale. She was the loudest of the team, and by far the most entertaining. She could make anyone laugh, and that's exactly what she did then too. She turned such a serious moment for me into just a casual, no big deal moment. Taylor had been right behind me the entire time, but I had done it, all by myself. And the team couldn't have been more accepting.

Throughout the high school season, the team grew closer and closer to each other, and Spale grew more and more protective over me because of my Alopecia. For example, almost every game, I had to deal with at least one ref approaching me, and asking me why exactly I was wearing a hat. Or if there was anything dangerous in it that would harm other players. Yeah, a piece of cloth over my head was sadly their main concern. I remember the first time a ref had asked why, I bluntly replied, "Um, because I have no hair. Okay?" He apologized and didn't even look at me the rest of the game.

As games continued, and questions kept arising, Spale began to get fed up with it, probably even more than I was. One game she saw a ref conversing with me, and from across the field she yelled, "Seriously?! Is he asking about it, Lesley?? I swear I'm gonna…" she went off into mumbling something she knew would get her in trouble. But her getting all worked up always made the refs chill out and back off. She intimidated them, and I didn't blame them one bit. The season flew by, faster than any of us could imagine. As one of the Level Three teams, our records definitely didn't match up to the higher teams; in fact we barely won any games. However, I loved the girls. Even if we were losing, we still tried to make the best of it.

Entering my sophomore year, I hesitated on playing again. But this time, I was going to try to wear my wig (my second one), instead of the beanie. I was still playing on my Rush league team, for Fall Season and Indoor Season. I played in both of those seasons after my freshman year with the school, and had finally tried out my wig. Surprisingly, I had no problem with it for those seasons. It stayed on just fine, even when I gently headered the ball. Even though both the hat and wig were vulnerable, especially when I played soccer, I felt much more comfortable wearing the wig. So that's what I decided to wear for sophomore tryouts.

For that year, tryouts were held on our new fields behind the school. The year before, they had limited the teams from playing on the fields, unless it was for important games. My dad had driven me around to the back parking lot, wished me luck, and drove off. It was so windy that week. Out of any week, of course, that week was going to be the windiest. And I'm not exaggerating; it was one of the windiest days I had ever spent outside.

Once again, the pressure was on. One thing that somewhat reassured me was the double-sided tape they made for wigs. You could stick one side to your scalp, and the other side would stick to the wig. It wasn't that sticky, obviously if one side was for your own skin, but it was another thing to try and help keep wigs in place. I had gotten the tape for when I would be doing something active, mainly soccer. So I made sure to wear those during tryouts that week.

I flew down the million stairs that led from the parking lot to the main field. Everyone looked like little ants from the top. I remember feeling so nervous, so out of my comfort zone, so afraid of what could happen. I prayed; I prayed to God that He'd guide me through these tryouts, and possibly make the wind stop. I needed that, and I needed Him. I finally got to the bottom, met up with a couple friends, and circled around the main Coach who was announcing the overall plans for the week. I was still freaked out by all of the older juniors and seniors. But at least I wasn't a "fresh freshman" this year. We got to pick our teams for the first day, so of course all of the known Varsity players got together, then most of the good JV players, and then random groups of friends for the other teams; I was in one of those.

The wind was picking up, more and more as we played. It didn't help that the intelligent landscape architects built the fields right in a valley, but there was nothing I could do about it. The whole time I was playing, I couldn't stop thinking about my wig falling off because of the crazy wind. And then I'd start thinking time was almost up, or the coaches hadn't seen that good pass I made, or what if I don't make a good team, and so on. It was ridiculous the way I was filling my mind up with so many other unimportant things when all I had to do was play some soccer.

After realizing my requests to God about the wind stopping weren't exactly going to follow through that day, I snapped out of it, and decided to go all out for the next play. I was playing somewhat of a left forward, even though my regular position is left wing. The ball was making its way up the field towards me, and I began making a run for a pass that I could use for a shot. I glimpsed at the defender I would be up against. Of course, she was one of the best defenders on the Varsity team, a senior that year. She was tall and pure muscle: kind of like a brick wall. Honestly, she scared the heck out of me. But I had already started my run, and I wasn't going to give up on this one. I waited for the pass, which finally came and was heading straight for the defender. I wanted the ball so bad though, so I knew I'd have to challenge her for it. The ball was partially in the air, coming towards us, both of us trying to position ourselves to receive it. We collided, and we collided hard.

The next thing I knew, I was laying on my back, flat on the grass. I remember feeling a sudden rush of cold wind hit my head. My wig had been knocked right off! I reached for the top of my head, hoping to find my "security blanket," but no luck. It was gone. Everything felt like it was in slow motion. I rolled my eyes, anticipating the chaotic scene that was about to happen once I got to my feet. I quickly stood up, jogged over to my wig about ten feet away, grabbed it off the grass and put it back on my head as best as I could. The girl I had collided with was still standing there. She stared at me, speechless, with her hands over her mouth. I didn't exactly know what to say to her without her saying something first.

I oddly smiled and said, "Sorry?" questioning why I would even say that. I guess I was thinking of saying sorry for going in for such a tackle, but no, it was more like saying sorry for putting you through that, having you see that happen, and don't feel bad about it, it wasn't your fault.

"Omigosh, no don't be sorry…it's okay, I mean I'm sorry…" she had trouble getting the words out, but I mean I don't know what I would have said either. We jogged back, closer to the center of the field where the ball was. To my surprise, none of the girls had really stopped playing, or stopped to watch. Just the girl I hit. I felt beyond embarrassed, and over exposed. "That was the last thing I had wanted to happen, and it did, awesome…" I thought to myself.

Tryouts were almost done anyway, so I held it together until the end. But inside, my emotions were tearing me up. I felt like disappearing. Just a snap of my fingers and bam, I'd be gone. But instead, I had to deal with fifteen minutes left of suffering. Once the coach had told us we could leave, I pulled my freshman year coach over, and told her I wouldn't be back for the rest of tryouts. I told her I was done, because of what had happened that day. She did her best to support me, but I could tell she was disappointed.

I sprinted up the stairs to my dad's car. I hopped in, trying to avoid the wind, and immediately started bawling. The only words I could get out to anyone were "my wig fell off…" and that's where I left it. I said it to my dad, my mom once I got home, and my best friends at the time, Catherine and Madi.

When I got home, my mom and Michelle (Catherine's mom) were sitting on the couch in the family room. My dad had called my mom on the way home from the school, and quickly told her what had happened. I didn't even notice him dialing, but apparently he did, and both moms knew about it when I stepped into the house. Before I could even say anything, Michelle rushed over to me and hugged me with all of her strength. She was such a petite, little woman, and I had always thought of her like that: but not then. She was more than just herself at that moment. And because of how big her heart was, it made her that much bigger and stronger. She held me as I cried into her shoulder. She kept whispering, "I'm so sorry sweetie, it's okay, I'm so sorry." The tone in her voice was the saddest I've ever heard her. She was always a loud and happy person, but not then.

After what was probably a good five minutes of hugging and crying, I told them I just wanted to go to my room alone for a little. I went upstairs, got in some warmer clothes, and wrapped myself up in blankets on my bed. I cried more. I cried until my pillow was soaked with tears. I drifted in and out of sleep, waiting for Madi and Catherine to rescue me.

The two of them had gotten there at different times, each so sympathetic and sorry for me. I told each of them the story, and asked what they thought I should do. I personally had no intention of going back to try-outs at that time. I was so against it. But after talking to my friends and parents, I slowly began to change my mind. They strongly encouraged me to go back. And I realized I couldn't just give up like that. It was so unlike me. I needed to prove to myself, my friends, my family, and everyone else who had seen what happened that I could come back from something like this. I needed to overcome that fear of embarrassment and the thought that everyone was thinking certain things when, really, they didn't care half as much as I did. Even if I wasn't going to play that season, I needed to at least finish another tryout day. That was the goal I set, and when I set goals, because of my determination, I'll meet them.

I went back to tryouts the next day and played my heart out. I remember my coach from freshman year frantically running up to me, so ecstatic to see me. She didn't think I'd come back. She hugged me and excitedly said, "I'm so happy you're here!"

"Yeah, me too," I said smiling.

I ended up not playing that year for high school. I figured I needed somewhat of a break from all of it, and I could focus on my academics. And I know I'd be playing in the fall for my League team. I don't regret not playing that year. What I do regret though is how I reacted when my wig fell off. I look back on it today and almost laugh. I wish I would have gotten up, grabbed my wig, ran it over to the coaches, handed it to them and said, "Can you hold this please?" and then kept playing. That's much, much more like me.

For You, Lord

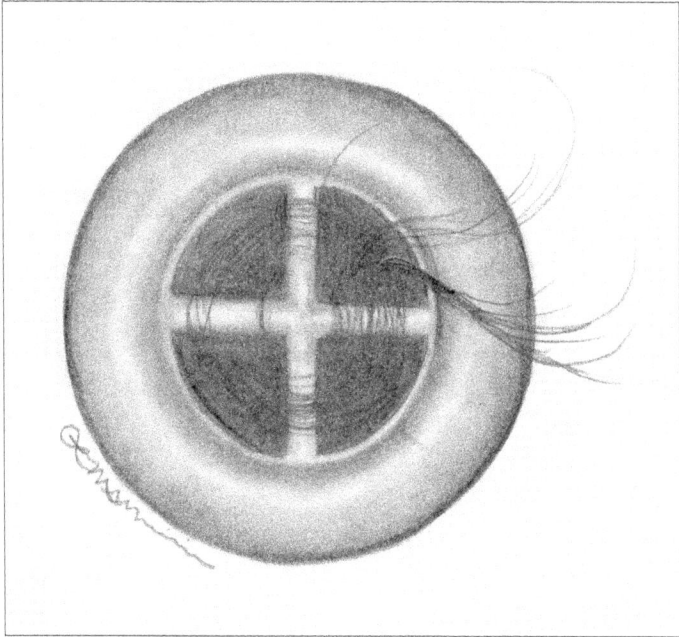

"I will never judge you by your looks. I will always love you for the sweet and wonderful girl you are on the inside."

~Mikkel B.

As I experienced and dealt with the effects of Alopecia, I was forced to approach everyday events in a much different way. You saw how I handled it with friends, school, and even soccer. I wasn't exactly satisfied with how some of those stories ended because, like I said before, that's not always like me. I usually handle things in a more positive manner instead of having some dramatic melt down.

For example, back in ninth grade when I wore a beanie for high school soccer, I specifically remember a practice that was inside. It was blizzarding in the middle of April—nothing out of the ordinary when you lived in Colorado. The fields were obviously in no condition to play on, so the coaches had decided soccer practice would be inside the school that day. Unfortunately, that most likely meant we'd be running through the halls the whole time because there was barely any space to do that elsewhere.

Once the final bell for school rang at 2:20, almost all of the students were cleared out in about ten or fifteen minutes. And that's about when soccer practice would start. So, I was never too afraid of running into someone when I had my beanie on because there would only be a few people wandering around in the commons area. And thankfully, I almost never knew them.

But on this lovely blizzard day, my team and I began jogging easily; pacing ourselves for the overall distance we'd be covering. A group of three guys I saw basically everyday in my classes were standing right by the vending machines. As we ran down a narrow hall, I could see ahead of us the three guys just goofing around. "Please don't know them, please don't know them," I thought to myself. When we passed them, of course they all had to turn around and stare at us—not like we look that good in soccer clothes, come on. I quickly glanced over to see if I knew them, and right then, one was looking straight at me. "Crap!" I thought, "I know them ALL, and they totally saw me!" I knew the boys well, but not well enough to the point where they knew about my Alopecia and my wig. I kept praying that they hadn't noticed it was me, but I knew they had.

The next day, during one of our passing periods, I was standing by my two good friends, Erica and Dylan. Suddenly, a boy jumped into our circle saying, "Hey!" It was one of the guys I had seen yesterday. He was Dylan's friend, so it wasn't strange for him to come over. We were all chatting normally when the kid started talking about hair. He started explaining how pretty he thought Erica's and mine were, because we both had dark, thick hair.

"Hey Lesley, you play soccer for the school right?"

"Yeah," I said.

"Okay that's what I thought…but I could have sworn I saw you running with the team yesterday, inside, and you were wearing like a beanie. I thought you were bald or something!"

Erica and Dylan froze up. I knew they wanted to stick up for me, but they had no idea what to do or say. I just smiled at him, trying to figure out how I would put this…

"I am bald, actually." I continued to smile.

"No you're not," the kid laughed, not believing it for one second.

"No, really, I am. This is a wig. And for soccer, I wear a beanie because it's easier." There was an awkward silence. I kept smiling to try and keep the situation as comfortable as it could be. He was so surprised, and I could see how bad he felt.

"Omigosh, I, I didn't know…"

"Oh it's okay! Really, I know you didn't know, I'm not mad or anything. It's fine!" People began hustling to their next class, anticipating the bell. We all knew we had to get to class, but I felt like I was the only one in command.

"Okay Erica, ready to go? Bye guys!" I said, nudging Erica to start moving with me. I didn't expect her or Dylan to do anything. They knew he wasn't intentionally trying to hurt my feelings, and I knew that too. That's why I wasn't upset at all, and that's exactly how I, the real me, would handle a situation like that. I stayed positive, told him it was okay, and went to class like nothing had happened.

Looking back on it, I just can't believe how much appearance matters to everyone, especially us teenagers. We're all so caught up in what we look like to other people when, really, the important thing is how we act and be ourselves in front of one another. With the whole "boys seeing me in a beanie" experience, I realized how, at first, I only cared about the appearance of it, and how a guy would suddenly see me without my long, dark hair. But once I was confronted with it, it was my attitude and reaction that would really matter. And fortunately, I handled it the best possible way I knew how.

People weren't going to judge me on the fact that I WAS bald; instead they'd judge me on how I dealt with BEING bald.

*   *   *

Ever since I could remember, I've been "boy crazy" as my mom likes to say. I remember even in kindergarten, taking the boy I had a crush on under the art table to kiss him. As I got older, especially in high school, I began wanting to seriously date people. I had always drooled over the fantasy love stories, wishing one day that could be me. And I enjoyed being in relationships; I liked having a guy as a best friend, always there for me and protecting me.

Freshman year, I met J.B. We met through church actually, and experienced Confirmation, one of the Catholic Seven Sacraments, together. During the Confirmation Retreat was when he and I really grew close and connected. After that though, I didn't see him much because we went to rivaling schools. But a year later, as sophomore year began, we started hanging out again. I had always kind of pictured him as a good friend, but I started to realize I liked him more than that.

As you already know, all of my hair fell out in December of freshman year. My doctors boosted me up on medications, and time was the only thing that would show progress. My hair slowly began growing back, pretty thin, but still dark black. It felt like it took forever, but eventually, by the summer before junior year, I had a full head of hair again. I've always been more comfortable with longer hair; however, I kind of liked it short for the time being. It was fun and flirty, and really easy to style; in fact I would just leave it how it was when I got out of the shower. Throughout the summer, I wore it short most of the time. As you can imagine, wearing a wig in hot weather is like wearing a whole other layer on your head. So my natural hair suited me best.

In the middle of July, Catherine, J.B., one of J.B.'s good friends, and I all went on a Church Retreat called Steubenville. It was in downtown Denver at the Convention Center. Our youth leaders had told us it was basically like the Confirmation Retreat, but ten times bigger and more inspirational. I remember being so excited; it was going to be like a reunion for all of us!

After arriving at our hotel, we quickly settled into our rooms (of course Catherine and I were roommates). The next morning, I had awakened earliest to take a shower first. As I washed my hair with shampoo, I felt it all over again. I felt my hair, slowly losing its grip on my scalp and getting wadded up into my hands. "You have got to be kidding me..." I thought. "It's all the way in! Why now?! I thought I had learned my lesson from this the first time!" I couldn't believe it. I was losing my hair for the second time. I had a gut feeling it wouldn't just be a couple of patches; for some reason I knew, deep down, that it would be all of it again. And it was going to happen fast, really fast.

I told Catherine and J.B. about it as soon as I got them somewhat isolated from our big church group later that day. We were on a pretty tight schedule, and a lot of other people were there so I didn't want anybody freaking out about it. They both did their best to reassure me that it might just be a little hair loss, nothing big, and that I should enjoy this Retreat while I could.

That day, a man got up to speak about saints, and very holy people. Towards the end of his presentation, he mentioned a teenage girl, Chiara Badano, who had bone cancer. She believed so deeply in God that she knew He had given a painful cancer to her for a reason, and loved Jesus as much as possible. Chiara died at 18 years old. But when she was going through chemotherapy, and began losing her hair, clump by clump, she would hold each handful and say, "For You, Lord." My heart stopped. God was showing me all of the signs. Once again, if I was going to lose all of my hair, He found the perfect place for me to be; I was surrounded by people that believed in Him and friends that loved me—with or without hair. "I need to do that," I thought.

The next morning, our last day there, I showered first again. Honestly, I was almost excited to try the technique the girl had done. I was as gentle as I could be on my scalp, slowly and carefully rubbing in shampoo. I took my hands down to see two handfuls of hair. I took a deep breath, closed my eyes, and said, "For You, Lord." I let go of the hair and let it drop to the drain. It felt so much more relaxing and calm when I said that. And from that day on, I promised myself that every handful of hair lost was for God Himself, and He had a plan for me.

Right after Steubenville, I was off on a two-week trip in Europe with my family. I had just discovered a bigger God in my own heart, and now I was going to see a bigger example of God's creation. We were going to see both Ireland and Italy. I was ECSTATIC. I had always been crazy about Europe, and now I was going to see the two countries of my background! I couldn't wait. However, I couldn't keep the thought from my mind that I was right in the process of losing my hair. I wasn't sure how this truth would affect my ability to enjoy my trip. Thankfully, I had a gorgeous wig we had bought at the beginning of summer, my fourth synthetic one, so that could help keep me safe and comfortable.

We stayed in various hotels while we were there. Each hotel had its own character, filled with the art and culture of the town we were visiting at the time. However, each hotel bathroom was just a reminder of having to take another shower. I can honestly say I left a part of me in every drain, literally. I continued to lose more and more hair. Every time though, I'd recite my line, "For You, Lord." It's what helped me let go, and move on to the rest of the spectacular days awaiting me. I wasn't about to let me losing some hair ruin this amazing trip of a lifetime. No, I wouldn't allow it to do that. Instead I stayed optimistic through the whole trip, and focused on a world I admired and loved.

When I was in Europe, J.B. and I did our best to email each other to stay in touch. Occasionally, I had the chance to get on a computer and the Internet at one of the hotels, so that's how we'd communicate. We missed each other quite a bit, and he was pretty much the only reason I wanted to come home.

After what was probably the two best weeks of my life, I finally arrived home. J.B. had actually been at my house a lot while I was gone; he and his dad had started working on painting my bathroom walls. I had wanted to re-do them that summer, and J.B. had offered to help, so they came over while we were away. Not only did they start the project, they totally re-did all the walls, and it looked amazing. I had a brand new bathroom to go along with my brand new point of view.

I couldn't wait to thank him the night I got to my house. He came over as soon as we were home. I gushed to him about how special the bathroom remodel was to me. I then tried telling him just a few of my favorite experiences in Europe, but there was so much to share! We were in my family room, and we updated each other on everything. He knew from Steubenville and the couple of emails I sent that I was losing my hair again. And he knew that it was a big part of my trip, even if I didn't say much about it.

"Lesley, I have kind of a surprise for you. Something I want to show you." I couldn't believe there was another surprise, the bathroom was enough and now he had something else.

"Okay, go for it." I said, anxiously waiting for what he was about to reveal.

"Alright…now I know this whole hair thing has been really hard for you. And losing your hair again must be one of the worst. But I think one of the hardest things about it is that you're doing it alone. That no one else has it that you know. So, I thought it might help if… if I had it too. I shaved some spots on my head for you." J.B. lifted some hair up and out of the way, making a small area of shaved hair visible to me. There were about four spots. I was speechless. He was so right; I had been doing so much of this alone. And as my boyfriend, he only wanted to experience it with me the best way he could. My eyes filled up with tears.

"J.B., omigosh, that's the sweetest thing anyone has ever done for me! Thank you, I can't believe you'd do that!" I gave him one of the biggest hugs, trying to show my appreciation for what he did.

His willingness to support what I was going through inspired me to ask one more favor of him. I had lost a majority of my hair in Europe, and barely had any left. To make it easier when losing it, I wanted to cut my remaining hair as short as possible, so it wasn't such a hassle in the shower like it had been before. I asked J.B. if he would help cut it. He accepted, and we settled down in front of the mirror. I handed him the scissors, and smiled at him in our reflection to help him feel more comfortable. I was suddenly reminded of when my mom had asked me to do this same thing for her all those years ago. And now I truly understood why she had smiled the entire way through.

Eventually, after about a year together, J.B. and I found our interests going opposite ways. We mutually agreed to just remain friends, but I will never forget the gift he gave to me that summer.

Early on, Alopecia attacked my confidence, day in and day out. First, having it in patches in middle school, I lost a lot of faith in myself, and generally tried staying away from having a "real boyfriend." But, when losing my hair completely for the first time, I changed my thought from, "omigosh, how will I still be pretty for the boys?" to, "how will I carry myself? How will I keep the confidence that boys see and appreciate in me?"

Because of my summer with J.B., I finally figured it out; I could use my disease to my advantage in one way at least. Alopecia was a part of me, and I couldn't help it or stop it no matter what I did. So whoever wanted to be with me would have to accept it, and accept me the way I was. It would show that a guy was looking at more than just my hair. It would show that he was interested in my whole personality. The way a boy reacted to it would flat out tell me if we could have a future together. I knew it wasn't just my hair that kept a guy liking me; it was much more than that. And the right boy would see straight through the disease, and accept me for me.

The Real Deal

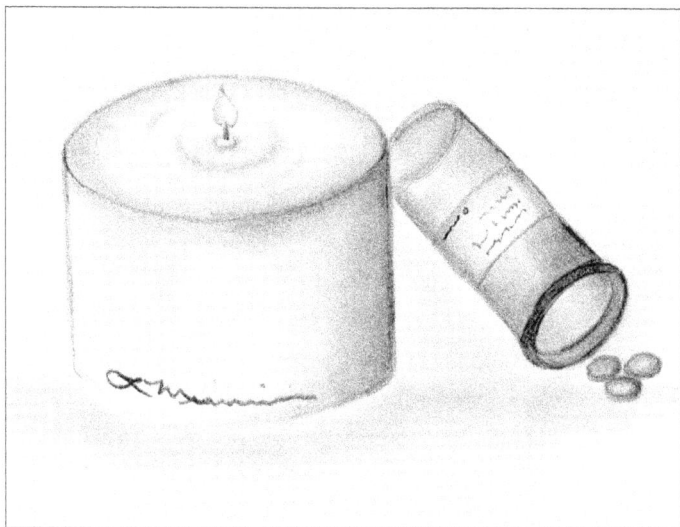

"Hi, beautiful girl. Until today, I had no idea about your disease. This shows how truly strong you are! You have really been able to overcome adversity. I now have even more respect for you than I did before."

~Darci A.

I've basically explained the social side of my life: school, friends, family, sports, and boys. But medically, my life was on a whole different page. Thankfully, Alopecia is not literally harmful to the body. However, certain medications and methods recommended for treatment always have their own side effects and risks.

With the first couple spots I had back in seventh grade, I would see Dr. S once a month and receive the Cortisone injections in my head. Those are very helpful because they get to the spots accurately, but that process still takes a while to start showing results of actual regrowth. The only real down side is obviously the pain, and small, temporary indentations to the scalp where the injections occurred.

As my spots continued to spread over my head, Dr. S suggested we needed something more powerful. We ended up discussing putting me on an oral steroid called Prednisone. I had been on Prednisone as a child, but only for my severe asthma. I have what they call a triad; this relates asthma, allergies, and eczema together. And fortunately, Prednisone can help pretty much all of those. It's a miraculous drug to most people, but some of its side effects can be the worst. It causes weight gain/increased appetite, varied emotions (mood swings), restlessness, increased sweating, and having trouble staying focused. And yes, I had all of those. Like I said, they can be the worst.

The one good side effect, though, was hair growth. Dr. S felt like if we were really going to kick this disease out completely, we needed to go all out: go big or go home, right? I was put on 80 milligrams a day as my starting point, and then would taper down each week until I was off of it. That's an extremely high dose for a young girl. And all of those side effects were just magnified for me. Within just a few weeks, I went from an athletic, thin build to gaining thirty pounds. My cheeks blew up, I was fighting with many of my friends due to the mood swings, I felt tired and useless, the sweating is self-explanatory, and my mom even had to write letters to my teachers explaining why I may not be as focused in class.

All of these led to some of the hardest and most embarrassing times of my junior high life. I didn't even realize how bad it all got until I was on a much lower dose and the side effects were fading. Even though the areas where I had lost hair began to grow back, only a month later after getting off of the pills completely, I began finding more spots again. It was sad to see it fail after all it had put me through.

Pushing Prednisone aside, they decided to try a Topical Acid Cream. Once again, the reason my hair falls out is because my white blood cells mistakenly read my hair follicles as something foreign, so they attack them causing hair loss. This is a huge mess up in my immune system, so a lot of the treatments work to try and restart healthy immunity. The Topical Acid Cream purposely gives you a small allergic reaction on your skin to try and somewhat jump-start your immune response. We tried the cream for only about a month, and I wanted off of it immediately. Once the cream was on, it felt like my scalp was slowly burning off. I overreacted to the allergic stimulation, and my scalp itched like crazy. I'd have open sores; they'd ooze, and then scab. My skin would get so tender and vulnerable that the last thing I wanted to do was touch it, but I had to in order to itch away the feeling for the time being. It was terrible and annoying, and I couldn't stand scratching my head that hard to the point where my skin was so damaged. It looked bad enough to Dr. S that she wanted to culture test it and send it to the lab just in case it was severely infected. And sadly, after using this method, we saw no major hair growth. Checked that one off the list.

After discovering my bad reaction with the Topical Acid Cream, we went back towards oral pills. Dr. S recommended Cyclosporine, a very strong medication with, once again, the side effect of hair growth. It also causes trembling and shaking in the hands, high blood pressure, more likelihood to bleed, and major kidney and liver problems. Yay… They warned me about being very cautious if I fell or cut myself because of the bleeding issue. They set me on a pretty average dose of Cyclosporine for a couple of months. Thankfully, the serious side effects were quite rare, and didn't seem to bother me. We saw good and fast hair growth too! It worked very well until I was off of it for about two months when suddenly my hair started falling out again. This was around the time when I lost ALL of my hair freshman year. Another fail.

Dr. S was running out of ideas; she was an amazing doctor, but now my Alopecia Totalis, instead of Areata, became more complicated and out of her reach. She had tried everything she was comfortable with, and her methods initially showed progress, but then failed to keep that once I was off of them. The last thing Dr. S had heard of was a treatment called PUVA light. It had recently just been reported how this light treatment had helped initiate hair growth, even in Alopecia patients. But she didn't know enough about it, so she suggested that we start seeing Dr. Norris, the Chief of Dermatology, and also a specialist in Alopecia, down in Aurora at the University of Colorado. She hoped he would have a good opinion on the PUVA light treatment.

Soon after working with Dr. S, we called Dr. Norris. He's one of the top dermatologists in the country, so for a first meeting, it took a while to get an appointment with him. I remember seeing him for the first time; he was an aged man, but one that just radiated wisdom when he walked into the room. He was more than experienced and had seen almost every type and form of Alopecia. He shook my hand firmly but in a gentle way, letting me know that he was here to help me, and he was determined to find a solution for this.

As we shared my history of hair loss cycles and past medications, you could see how intrigued he was by Alopecia; he had a passion for helping individuals with the disease, and he clearly only wanted to find a cure. After being updated on everything I had experienced so far, Dr. Norris took his time to soak up all of the information. He was careful with his words and his thoughtful suggestions. And once it was said, he backed it up 100 percent. I admired his confidence like that, and it only made me trust him more.

Hearing my story and relating it to so many other similar patients, Dr. Norris decided to start me on the combination of Prednisone and Methotrexate: both pills. The reason why he wasn't in favor of the PUVA treatment was because he personally hadn't seen that much success with it, and if it was effective, it was only on people who were completely bald. At the time, I had some very thin patches wanting to grow back (nothing that looked promising), so that hair makes it hard for the light to get to the scalp correctly.

Anyway, I already knew about Prednisone, but Methotrexate was something new to me. Methotrexate is often used on arthritis patients. Its side effects are somewhat similar to Cyclosporine; it causes drowsiness and is very toxic to the kidney and mainly the liver. It's required to get your blood drawn frequently while on this medication because the doctors have to monitor it well and watch for any sudden changes. That didn't faze me; I was so used to needles by this point because I had gotten shots often as a kid for the triad condition. I had experienced shots in my head, and had gotten my blood drawn many times before.

We agreed to the combination of pills, and trusted Dr. Norris because he had seen lots of hair growth when using the two together. I made it very clear that I would NOT go on a high dose of Prednisone again just because of my previous experience. The highest I would go was ten milligrams a day, and Dr. Norris was fine with that; that's about all he needed. It's the Methotrexate that I would try on a higher dose.

I spent about two and a half years on this medication plan. While I was on it, I definitely saw some positive results, but I couldn't stay on it forever. According to Dr. Norris, I had reached the maximum dosage for liver safety. And, as soon as they took me off, I slowly began losing my hair again.

We continue to see Dr. Norris for regular check-ups and eagerly await new procedures that may show promise for long term success. And maybe even a cure…

*   *   *

But wait! There's more! I know you want to hear about my wig escapades. I had gone through four synthetic wigs up until the end of junior year. After getting my first wig at the place in Cherry Creek, we decided to check out the other store my mom had thought of for all of our other purchases; that was Hana's place. And the main person who helped me through my wig decisions was Hana. Like my mom, Hana's story was that she had survived breast cancer, and gone through chemotherapy. She experienced losing all of her hair at once, and couldn't help but notice that there weren't many options for those who needed wigs or hair appliances. And she was committed to change that by opening up her own store, Hana Designs.

Hana Designs is one of the most calming places I've ever been. The energy it gives off is just soothing and subtle. The outside world gets quiet and silent, and it's like only that store exists. It smells incredible because candles are always lit and radiating their aromas. It just feels fresh to me, like a new beginning every time I enter. To the right all the wigs are displayed, and to the left is her desk and a few hair-cutting stations. Also on the left are a few aisles filled with other hair products and supplies. I feel the most beautiful when I'm there because nothing else seems to matter, and it's where Hana and any other client would immediately accept me.

Hana is probably one of the cutest, sweetest adults I have ever seen and met. She's a very pretty, small, Asian woman who carries herself much bigger than you'd expect. Now that she has her hair back and embraces it so much more, she likes to play around with it; for example, she's had her hair completely bleach blonde before and still looked absolutely adorable!

I learned everything I know about wigs just from her. She's seen quite a bit of Alopecia kids, but I think (or hope) I stand out to her. She always mentions how strong I am for going through this, and also how well I take care of my wigs. A synthetic wig that's supposed to last about three months I could carry out for nine. Once I purchased a wig, I just cherished it, and took care of it like it was really my own hair. I learned how to wash it best once a week, how to style it in various ways, and even curl my synthetic wigs with hot curlers. Curlers weren't like curling irons, so the hair wouldn't sizzle. Take that, Barbie™!

I had always thought about getting a real hair wig, even though I was completely satisfied with my synthetic wigs. They weren't as much work because you didn't have to wash them as frequently, and the style on a synthetic wig stayed the same. But, after a while, I started to want the real deal; I wanted to be able to curl it and straighten it and have it look and feel like real hair. I just wanted that kind of sensation back, because honestly, I missed it. I talked to my parents about it, and they were so proud with how I handled the synthetic wigs that they were sure I could do just the same with a real hair wig. Plus, the great thing about genuine hair is that it lasts for more like three years instead of three months. The only thing in my way was the price.

We knew we could trust Hana, so we asked for her opinion as well. We really wanted our insurance to be able to cover a majority of the price, if not all, but the answer we received was that "a wig is considered a beau-

ty product, so we'll be able to cover $150.00 dollars."
"Are you kidding me?" I thought. Might as well not cover anything if you think $150.00 dollars will really help when it comes to a wig costing much more than two thousand dollars. My mom and I planned on writing to the insurance company trying to fight our point that it was much more than a beauty product, but we couldn't really find the chance and time; at least not for this wig.

For a real hair wig, there are three main types ranging in coarseness: Asian hair, Indian hair, and European hair. Asian is the thickest and least expensive, European the thinnest and most expensive. Also, the longer the wig is, the more money because it's asking for more hair. Hana suggested European hair would be the best because it was the most like my normal hair (coming from a European background).

Hana hooked us up with one of the most gorgeous wigs I'd seen. My mom and I went into her store for me to check it out and try it on. The moment I saw it I knew it was for me; and I loved it! It was jet black, there was a lot of it, and it was wavy when it got wet, just like mine used to be. The wave was perfect, the length was perfect, it just needed to be thinned out and styled a bit. I couldn't believe how much it resembled my own hair. Both my mom and Hana approved right away, and knew it was exactly what we were looking for. Hana pulled some strings to give us the best price and discount she could, but because it was so long and it was European, it came out to be about $3500.00 dollars.

Walking out of there with my new purchase was one of the best feelings in the world. I couldn't help but feel guilty, though... I knew how much money we had just spent, I mean it was like half the price of my car! I felt like that was too much to spend on hair. But when I expressed my concern to my mom, her response was, "Lesley, this is what I do and you don't need to worry about this one at all. I'm the mom here, it's okay. Besides, this is more than just hair to you." She was right, again. This new wig represented a more honest expression of me. I couldn't help but smile the whole way home.

Now it was time to see Dawn for some style.

It's Okay, Everything's Okay

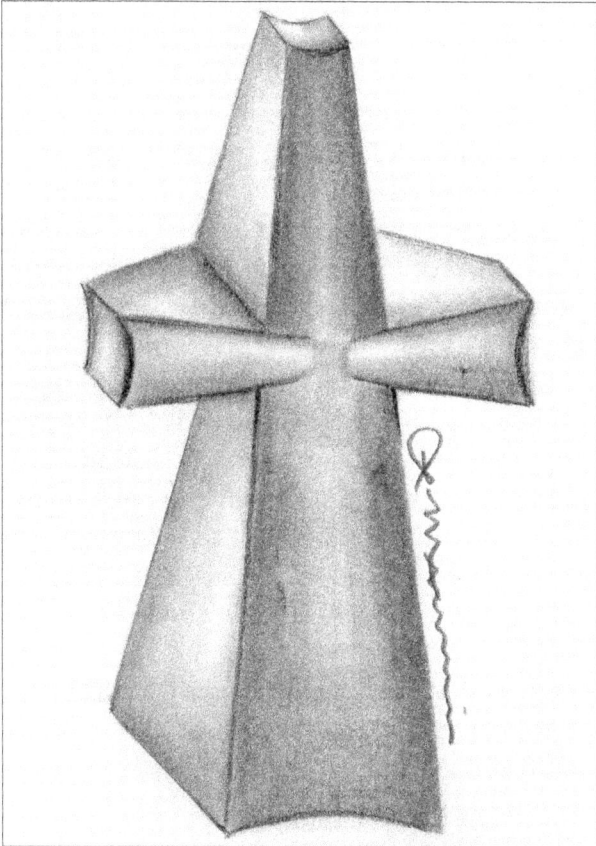

"God isn't putting us through all of this so that we can keep it to ourselves. He does it so we can share what we've learned with others and give them strength through our suffering."

~Shannon K.

I stepped into Dawn's lovely new salon that had just opened up. Since I started seeing her for my haircuts, she had been in three places. This one, though, was even closer to home, and she started work there with all of her good friends. I knew she'd be sad to hear I had lost all of my hair, AGAIN, but I was still beyond excited to see her, just for our traditional updates.

I had my fourth synthetic wig on, with my new real hair wig in a box for her to cut this time. As soon as she saw me, she rushed over to say a big hello like always. She walked me back to her station and sat me down in the black, wide chair. She asked what we'd be doing today, exactly, and what the whole scoop was on the hair. My cheerful grin suddenly turned upside down and I could tell she sensed what had happened.

"I lost it again, Dawn. When we were in Europe for our trip…but really it's over with now. I mean, I've been through it so many times, I'm honestly used to it. Like, of course I'm sad, but seriously, I can't be upset about it forever. With the wigs now and everything, I'm just able to kind of deal with it all. It doesn't bother me as much anymore."

"Aw, Lesley, I'm so sorry. I can't believe, though, how hard it would be to lose it all again, completely, after you had it all back for the summer. That's got to be tough, girl."

"Well yeah, definitely, it was. Especially after I was convinced it was in for good. But really I've just gotten to the point where I'm over it. This disease obviously won't make up its mind, and is simply going to be a part of me for a while it looks like. I try not to look at it as such an awful thing anymore, but more of a blessing.

Because look how much it's taught me and made me stronger, ya know?"

"Exactly, I completely agree with you, sweetie, that you have this for a reason. You are so much stronger now because of this. You have this whole other perspective on life that kids and teens your age may never go through. You see things now with so much more appreciation and importance. You get that hair isn't everything. It's only looks. You get that now, and you see what really matters in life. You're right to look at this in a positive way, as a blessing, Les, because you know what I think? I think that God gave you this for a reason. Alopecia keeps coming back because I think He's telling you you need to do something about it. Like... writing a book on this. Yes, that's it. I think you should write a book!"

"Omigosh, Dawn, I'd love to do something like that! But that'd be impossible to do while I'm still in high school, with all the homework, and classes, and soccer and stuff. I could never find the time for that. And how would it ever get made or published or whatever?"

"No, Lesley, really! I know this woman! She's an author herself but is also a co-author. She helps people write these incredible stories, ones like yours. And she's not in it for the money or anything; it's all about getting these stories out and on paper. I know she'd be so interested! You'd love her!"

"Really?! How do you know her, exactly?"

"I cut her hair, too. In fact, I think she's coming in this week. I'll give her your number, and you can call her whenever and try to meet up or something! And I'll let her know, when I see her, what we have in mind. Would you consider doing that?"

"Well, yeah! I would. I mean if she'd be there to help edit and format and really make it an actual book, I'll definitely try!"

"Okay, perfect. I'll let her know. And remind me to get her number before you leave. Okay, now let's talk about possible chapters…"

*   *   *

Dawn was completely right. My Alopecia disease was a blessing—a gift from God. Alopecia chose me because it's what God wanted. From the very beginning, He had a plan. He knew how much I'd struggle, how much I'd cry, how much I'd blame Him for this. He knew all of that. But He also knew that out of so many kids, I was the one who could go through it, and actually overcome it. I've always been an extremely motivated and determined girl, so God knew I'd strive for something positive out of this.

I have this disease so I'm capable of truly opening up my eyes to the world. I am able to see the important things in life. When I meet people now, my initial reaction isn't to observe their appearance: how skinny, how curvy, how tan, how pale, how short, how tall, how muscular, or how thin. None of that really matters to me anymore. It's crazy to think how those aspects are what certain people revolve their lives around. They're missing out on such a big picture. As cliché as it sounds, it really is what's on the inside, not the outside. That's what matters, and that's what makes someone who he/she is. Am I just a girl with no hair who wears a wig? No. I'm a girl who can carry herself high, with confidence and faith in herself. I'm a girl who loves to love, help, and be

around people who accept me. And if they don't, then that's their problem, not mine; I've already found my solution.

I see everyone from a new perspective because of my Alopecia experience. I try to not look at WHAT people have done, but WHY they have done it, and HOW they handled it. Because that's exactly how I want and hope people view me. And we treat others like we want to be treated, right? I have taught myself to find the best in people. I know that every individual is capable of being the best person they can be. However, a majority of people haven't accomplished that. In fact, I haven't fully achieved it, but I, at least, know who my best person is and what she looks like. And because I've experienced it, I only hope to witness it in several other lives.

Now, I am so thankful for what Alopecia has put me through. Because without it, without the severe ups and downs of all of it, I would not be who I am today. I am Lesley Minervini, and I have Alopecia. I have the most supportive, loving, and caring family in the world. They're what I come home to. My brother challenges me and helps strengthen my overall character. My dad provides a quiet stability that ensures that we all feel safe when it seems like the world is falling apart. And my mom offers a special compassion for my situation because she personally experienced losing her hair. As you already know, even before I lost my first strand, she had taught me that beauty is how you choose to define it, "milky pens" and all.

I'm honored to have the most incredible friends anyone could ever ask for. And I'm not exaggerating. Every single one of them has gone out of their way to simply check up on me, see how things are going, offer to talk, respect my boundaries, but stay right by my side. Not one of them has let me down. They've been my backbone through all of this. To you, I say thank you with all of my heart.

This book, my story, and the lessons I've learned are for almost everyone. It's especially here for the ones going through hair loss. I want those dealing with Alopecia to know that, "What if we don't ever get our hair back? That's okay! Who cares! We're still the exact same people either way, with or without hair! We're not alone." This is for cancer patients, too. For those who are about to start, or are already in the process of, chemotherapy, this is to show you that you can and will get through the hair loss. If I did it with Alopecia, each and every one of you can definitely do it with cancer. For all the parents who would give literally anything to put themselves in their child's position, it's okay. They're going to get through it one way or the other. Even if that means they survive to stay with you, or leave to watch over you.

For all the people who think they don't relate to this, think again. You all have your struggles and insecurities. And each one of you has at least ONE positive thing you can pull out of those. Once you find it, just expand on it, let it overrule the negatives, and live your life to the fullest. Share it with others and encourage them to do the same.

I never thought that, as a high school student, I'd be writing an entire book. But I took the chance and look what came of it. We've been able to share my experiences together, and I hope I've helped you truly realize how valuable you are. My one last thing to share with you is a special event that took place at my church while I was praying. I usually had a list prepared in my mind of whom to pray for, but something told me to stop thinking so much and just let this moment be. It wasn't something that happened every day; this time it was much more personal and inspiring. And that's exactly why I end the book with this, because I only hope it inspires you too. God bless.

*   *   *

The Adoration

Saint Francis Cabrini Catholic Church
August of 2009

I drifted to somewhere so far away; it almost felt like it was out of this world. I didn't know where I was, but I was okay with that. I was outside, surrounded by absolutely nothing. As I slowly turned and turned again, a few things began forming. I felt soft, hot sand underneath my bare feet. I sank into it just a little, to the point where my toes weren't visible anymore. I wiggled them slightly just to feel the great sensation between each toe. Where was I? At the beach or something?

I peered up into the beaming sun that suddenly appeared. It was shining down stronger than ever, right down on me. It was warm, and the wind blew, but only at me. I felt the cool air hit my face but it was so soothing, so pleasant, that I didn't turn away. The air smelled dry. To my right, a slight hill was there with nothing on it. It looked like a desert now—just a pure golden blanket of sand with nothing to disturb it.

I sensed someone there, next to me and I finally turned around to see. It was Jesus Himself. He stood there, looking like all of the pictures I've seen of Him. But for some reason, I wasn't shocked at all. It's like I knew He'd be there. He smiled continuously, but didn't say anything. I just smiled back at Him. He grabbed my hand, and directed me to wherever He was taking me. I noticed, as we walked, He never walked in front or behind me, just directly next to me.

We were in no rush, so we took our time. There was still nothing in sight for miles, from what I could see at least, but the sand alone was just as beautiful. I was content just being with Him even though no words had been spoken yet. I looked over at Jesus. He wore a long, off-white cloak, like you see in most pictures. There was a thin rope tied around his waist to keep the cloak from dragging on the ground. His tan skin blended with the color of the sand. It seemed like He was glowing, even more than me, with the sun still beaming down on us.

After what felt like several minutes, Jesus finally stopped. He stopped walking so I did, too. He was looking in front of us, and I eventually looked up to see a small pond of the clearest water ever. It was in the middle of complete nowhere; this tiny pool of water just randomly appeared in the desert. There were a couple of green shrubs surrounding the water, but they left the overall attention to the pond. "How did this get here?" I first thought. But I didn't care; it was there for a reason obviously.

Jesus knelt down right next to the edge of the water. I did the exact same thing, knowing that I was one of his followers. He barely touched the water, almost testing it for something. He then cupped both hands slightly below the surface, and brought up a handful of water to His mouth. He looked over at me to give His approval that I could drink also. I did, following His exact motions. It tasted refreshing and cold to my warm lips and body.

Once I was done, I glanced over at Him, waiting to see what we were about to do next. But instead, He pointed to the water in front of me, signaling for me to look. I looked at my reflection. "Nothing too special," I thought. Jesus then gently held my face with both hands, turning my head towards Him. He gazed into my eyes and then, slowly, moved His hands to my hair. I hadn't realized it until then, but I had my wig on. He grabbed each edge of the wig and slowly pulled it off. He kissed my forehead and said His first words to me,

"It's okay," He smiled. He motioned for me to look again into the water. This time I took a deep breath, and peered into the water, recognizing my reflection again. But this time, I had a bald head with a couple patchy areas. It doesn't sound beautiful but it was. I felt the prettiest I ever had in my entire life. I stared at myself for a while, observing every detail on my face and head. "It is okay," I thought to myself. "I'm gorgeous the way I am. This is my blessing, my future. This makes me *me*. And that's okay. Everything's okay."

If you've been inspired or would like to add to the discussion presented in this book, please join the "Falling Out" community on Facebook at:

Search: Falling Out by Lesley Minervini

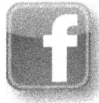

If you would like to contact Lesley directly about speaking engagements or more information, please contact her through Facebook.

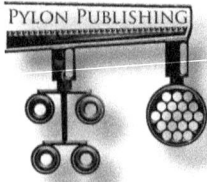

Are you an aspiring Author?

Getting published shouldn't be a dream.

Pylon Publishing LLC specializes in the publication of experienced and aspiring authors alike. The small and knowledgeable company can provide the most custom and specialized services necessary to turn your manuscript into a book quickly. Since Pylon Publishing works directly with the word's largest wholesale book distributor, Ingram Book Company, clients can feel at ease with the widest distribution - Amazon, Barnes and Noble, etc.

It is Pylon Publishing's goal and mission to give authors the most flexibility, distribution, and earnings for their work. As a result, every author retains full control of their book upon publication.

That's the Pylon Promise!